BENEATH THE
CORTICAL SURFACE

Beneath the Cortical Surface

Edison K. Miyawaki, M.D.

Copyright © 2020 by Edison K. Miyawaki, M.D.

Library of Congress Control Number:		2020911773
ISBN:	Hardcover	978-1-9845-8569-1
	Softcover	978-1-9845-8568-4
	eBook	978-1-9845-8567-7

All rights reserved. No part of this book may be reproduced or transmitted in any form or by any means, electronic or mechanical, including photocopying, recording, or by any information storage and retrieval system, without permission in writing from the copyright owner.

Any people depicted in stock imagery provided by Getty Images are models, and such images are being used for illustrative purposes only. Certain stock imagery © Getty Images.

Print information available on the last page.

Rev. date: 06/27/2020

To order additional copies of this book, contact:
Xlibris
1-888-795-4274
www.Xlibris.com
Orders@Xlibris.com

815937

Contents

1. Introduction: Proposal for a Seminar 1
2. *Ansa lenticularis* 3
3. Bed Nuclei of the *Stria Terminalis* 6
4. Claustrum 12
5. Diencephalon, embryology of 16
6. Eminences 22
7. Forebrain, caudal 26
8. *Globus Pallidus*, lateral (in particular) 29
9. Habenula 33
10. Infundibulum 36
11. Juxtallocortical Connection (to Hypothalamus) 39
12. *Kern* 43
13. Labeled Line 46
14. Macro-, Microcircuitry 52
15. *Nucleus accumbens septi* 57
16. Olfactory Tubercle 60
17. Projections of the Striasomal System 64
18. Quadrilateral Space of Broca 68
19. Reticular Nucleus of Thalamus 72
20. Sequences 76
21. Thalamocortex 79
22. Uncrossed? 88
23. Vascular Organ of the *Lamina Terminalis* 93
24. Wakefulness 98
25. X and Y relay cells 103
26. *Zona incerta* 108
27. The Themes of this Monograph 113

References 125

1.

Introduction: Proposal for a Seminar

I envision four to six participants for any given six-week period. The target audience would be those who've been exposed to introductory neuroanatomy, and who remain interested in the subject. Attendance in person is preferred—strike that, it will be mandatory. I write in 2020, in the midst of a viral pandemic that started in 2019, so I'll add that masks will be available and social distance maintained, assuming that we have real classrooms in the future.

Laptops and muted smart phones are permitted, provided that they don't impede communication with those present.

Beepers are categorically disallowed.

Each week, there's a preliminary assignment, to read a monograph. The reading only encourages each person to choose some aspect from that reading to explore *for the group*. Sessions, two-ish hours in length, happen once weekly. Thursdays in Boston's pre-solstice winter would be best, in the afternoon, when the sun sets early.

Everybody presents every week, save for one person. He, the seminar's organizer, has authored the monographs, and is present as a recording secretary for ideas or criticisms raised. The little books are: *The Crossed Organization of Brains*, *The Frontal Brain and Language*, *Learning the Brainstem*, *Teaching Hippocampal Anatomy*, *The Visual Cortices*, and a sixth, which you have in front of you.

*

The problem with my alphabetically organized list in this book is caprice. Why choose "*ansa lenticularis*" for A and "*zona incerta*" for Z; aren't the choices arbitrary? Yes, . . . but they aren't altogether random. Previously, I've written by in large about cortex, except for my short text–not a textbook in the least–on the brainstem.

In what follows, I talk about alphabetically arranged topics (all having to do with subcortical structures excepting brainstem) which interest me, perhaps you as well. You might think that I provide just an idiosyncratic dictionary through which you flip at random (you could do this), but you could also read the chapters in order to glean an attempted, continuous line of thought.

The spirit of the seminar applies to what follows. No one should expect encyclopedic performance. Brain anatomy deflates such aspirations, anyway.

*

As always in what I write or teach, errors of commission and omission are entirely my responsibility.

2.

Ansa lenticularis

We're familiar with the fact that a major output nucleus from the basal ganglia is the **medial**–or **"internal"**–*globus pallidus* (I'll refer to it as **medial GP**). Its output is to thalamus. Medial GP (as well as lateral GP) neurons are inhibitory with GABA as their major neurotransmitter.

What route(s) do medial GP axons take toward thalamus?

Several years ago, I finally found a diagram with just enough detail regarding the very crowded anatomy below thalamus (Haubenberger and Hallett, 2018; reproduced with permission). It's a cartoon of a coronal section, at a point along the anterior-posterior axis probably close to posterior commissure–in other words, behind the midpoint between **anterior and posterior commissures**.

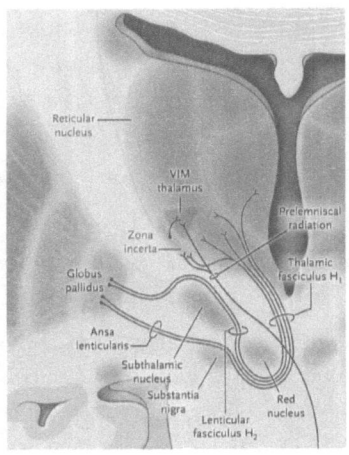

Medial GP is most medial aspect of the so-called **lentiform nucleus**. Medial GP is bounded superiorly and inferiorly by white matter, and its lateral border is an **internal medullary lamina of** *globus pallidus*, not marked by name in the diagram.

In 1895, Russian-Swiss neuropathologist Constantin von Monakow described (Nauta and Mehler, 1966) how a mass of fibers arising from medial GP cuts across the cerebral peduncle to form what he called *eine schlinge* (a sling); the Latin word *ansa* more tamely refers to a handle or a loop. A sling around what?

It appears that fibers sling around red nucleus, at least.

Enter another Swiss neuroanatomist, August-Henri Forel, who, in 1877 (Neudorfer and Maarouf, 2017), described three tegmental *fields*, all in the vicinity of red nucleus in the midbrain tegmentum. Forel thought that fibers originating from red nucleus formed a prerubral field or cap ("**H**") that either extends dorsally (as "**H1**") or ventrally (as "**H2**") around red nucleus. "H" abbreviates the German word *haube*, which is a cap or bonnet.[1]

Forel's nomenclature lingers to this day.

Von Monakow drew particular attention to a bifurcation depicted in the figure, a fork in the road that essentially starts at medial GP.

There's a *fasciculus lenticularis* or **lenticular fasciculus** (Forel field H2), that forms the dorsal capsule of the **subthalamic nucleus of Luys**.[2]

Then there's the *ansa lenticularis* in the literal sense of the term (in German, *linsenkernschlinge* or lens-nucleus-sling). The ansa forms a white-matter layer on the ventral edge of medial GP; its fibers pass across descending axons of the internal capsule, then they sling around red nucleus to join, along with fibers of the lenticular fasciculus, a **thalamic fasciculus** (Forel field H1) that heads superiorly to thalamus.

Note a curious projection whose origin is not indicated in the diagram: a line at the lower right-hand corner also projects towards thalamus; it decussates in the midbrain tegmentum. Called a **prelemniscal radiation**,

---

[1] There are, by the way, neurons in the fields of Forel which are given the name of a ***nucleus campi Foreli*** (Nauta and Mehler, 1966).

[2] Von Monakow also noted a "subthalamic fasciculus" that perforates across cerebral peduncle, ventral to the lenticular fasciculus, to enter subthalamic nucleus of Luys (Nauta and Mehler, 1966). We concentrate on lenticular fasciculus and ansa lenticularis.

its origin is a deep cerebellar nucleus (dentate), according to Haubenberger and Hallett; it is "pre-lemniscal" insofar as it is superior/anterior to medial lemniscus, which is present (but not represented in the diagram) in the area of the thalamic fasciculus (Forel field H1). The authors include the structure, because they highlight subthalamic and thalamic structures relevant to neurosurgeries for tremor and other movement disorders.

My intent in reproducing their useful and clear diagram is simpler. All I want to observe is that *ansa lenticularis*, lenticular fasciculus (Forel field H1), and the thalamic fasciculus (Forel field H2) are inhibitory, unidirectional projections (Haber, 2016).

I think inhibition and disinhibition (depending on striatal and other input to medial GP) of diencephalic thalamus is interesting, as we'll continue to explore in the next letter of the alphabet.

3.

Bed Nuclei of the *Stria Terminalis*

It's not the greatest advertisement, but at least the author is honest (Dumont, 2009):

> What exactly is this bed nucleus of the stria terminalis? This is a question that I, and possibly all of my colleague neuroscientists with interest in this region of the brain, get on a regular basis. Unfortunately, the simplest questions are often the most difficult to answer.

Firstly, what's in a name? Researchers have failed to reach consensus on whether "BST" or "BNST" is the most effective acronym for their structure of interest. . . . To our chagrin, both will probably continue to be commonly used. A description of BST (sic) [the author obviously prefers "BNST"] should start by reporting that it is a cluster of about 12 nuclei surrounding the caudal part of the anterior commissure, deep in the cerebral hemispheres.

The bed nuclei, part of what has been termed an "extended" amygdala (De Olmos and Heimer, 1999), are "at one extremity" (that's Dumont's phrase, used elsewhere in his paper) of the *stria terminalis*, which, I've taught in class, is a long fiber tract that passes from amygdala *posteriorly*, tucked in the nook-like, medial border between body of caudate and thalamus; then it loops forward to dive ventrally in the direction of anterior commissure, and it ends in structures near that commissure, particularly **septal nuclei** and hypothalamus.

But what's the meaning of "extended" or "at one extremity"? Are the bed nuclei of the stria terminalis *not* part of amygdala *itself*?

*

It's not easy, by the way, to visualize the stria terminalis, but one trick is to look for a **"terminal vein"**[3] also located in the nook between caudate and thalamus (the coronal image is at the level of amygdala):

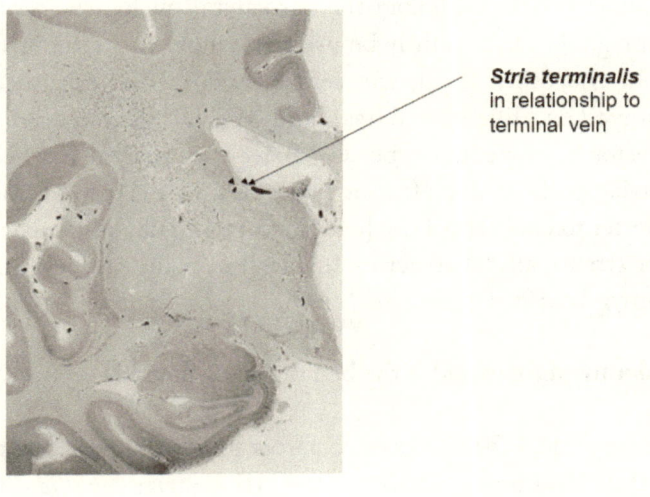

Stria terminalis in relationship to terminal vein

*

Back to our question: Are the bed nuclei of the stria terminalis *not* part of amygdala *itself*?

Turns out, the answer isn't straightforward, . . . *but it can be summarized briefly*. I'll borrow from McDonald (2003), who echoes the observations of Carl Burdach in 1822 that amygdala consists, very basically, of two components:

a **corticobasolateral amygdala**
and
a **centromedial extended amygdala.**

---

[3] Also known as the **superior (or anterior) thalamostriate vein**, it drains to internal cerebral vein, thence to the great cerebral vein (of Galen).

Then McDonald launches forth:

> The former appears to be a cortical-like sensory interface of the amygdala that is capable of associating information from different sensory modalities with each other as well as with their positive and negative emotional/behavioral valences. Because this unique function is associated with [corticobasolateral amygdala], and since Burdach used the amygdala to denote the basolateral nuclei, the term amygdala can certainly be used to denote this structure. On the other hand, the central and medial extended amygdala, like the dorsal and ventral striatopallidal systems, appear to be GABA-ergic striatal-like or striatopallidal-like effector structures. . . . [I]t might be better to conceive of the [extended amygdala] as a striatal or striatopallidal structure involved in many, but not all, amygdalar functions.

Extended amygdala includes the bed nuclei of the *stria terminalis*.

Swanson (2003, 2012c) goes so far as to say that the bed nuclei *are pallidal,* thus evoking a notion that cortico-striatal-*pallidal*-thalamo-cortical organization applies to amygdalar function. De Olmos and Heimer (1999) don't agree with Swanson, it should be said, because a closed cortex-to-cortex loop is not what they intended to demonstrate when they introduced the concept of an extended amygdala in the first place.

*

Looking at any image of amygdala, but especially when one finds Burdach's original from 1822, one wonders whether amygdala (almond nucleus or *mandelkern* in German) looks cortical:

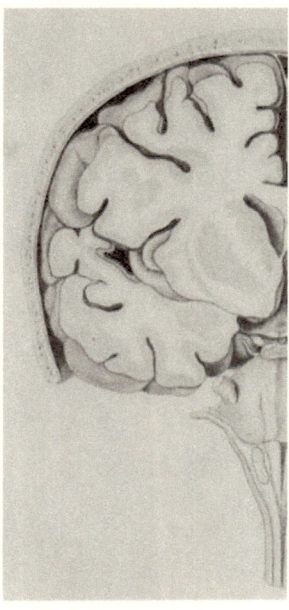 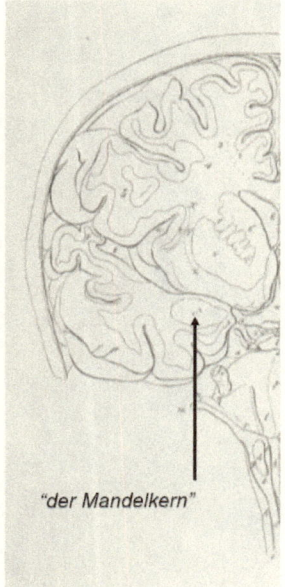

"der Mandelkern"

Burdach's schematic, to the right, doesn't indicate the wisps of grey matter inferior and medial to the almond in the unlabelled drawing. I learned years ago (Carpenter and Sutin, 1983) about a **periamygdaloid area** that technically is part of rhinencephalon, the latter also known as paleocortex. I think the wisps of grey are periamygdaloid cortex. Certainly a part of the amygdaloid complex is pallial (not pallidal)–viz., paleocortical, but not therefore neocortical.

The bed nuclei are what Swanson would collectively call a cerebral nucleus akin to caudate, putamen, or the medial or lateral *globus pallidus*, as opposed to cerebral cortex (Swanson, 2012c). But where's the actual bed of the nuclei of *stria terminalis*? Follow anterior commissure to its caudal extent. In standard sections, you don't visualize at a glance the curve in three dimensions that anterior commissure takes, but Longet (1842) helps us:

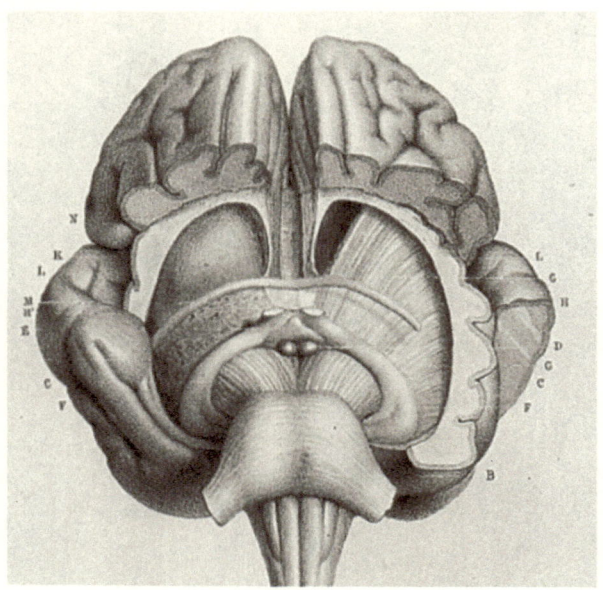

I won't mar the drawing by superimposing arrows on it. Let's just describe what the artist depicts. In the left hemisphere, to the right of the image, there's a relationship between the descending fibers of the *corona radiata* and the anterior commissure as the latter passes posteriorly/caudally. In the right brain, those descending coronal fibers aren't shown, so we can appreciate a relationship between the caudate head and the rostral anterior commissure. More posteriorly, the anterior commissure extends inferiorly, and traverses lentiform nucleus (both putamen and rostral *globus pallidus*).

The two main points, however, are:

1. anterior commissure's most caudal and lateral aspect brings it close to uncus and, within uncus, to amygdala; that caudal and lateral aspect also points to the bed nuclei; a good number of the nuclei are just dorsal to uncus, if you stain for them. Then, note also that...
2. deep to anterior commissure are *ventral* striatal and pallidal structures. If the drawing included them, they would emerge from the plane of the page towards your eyes.

As with *ansa lenticularis*, output from the bed nuclei relates to the interaction between telencephalon, including some but not all parts of amygdala, and diencephalon (especially, but not exclusively, the medial thalamus).

Back to McDonald (2003), who is so matter of fact that one feels an urge to thank him personally for clarity:

> The cerebral hemispheres consist largely of two major macrostructures: (1) cortical regions characterized by glutamatergic principle neurons and (2) striatopallidal regions characterized by GABAergic principal neurons. Specific portions of these macrostructures are connected to form functionally specific corticostriatopallidal circuits.

With respect to the striatopallidal aspect of the amygdaloid complex, he adds:

> It is tempting to speculate that the projections of the central and medial amygdalar nuclei [viz., the "centromedial" ones] to the *midline thalamic nuclei* might subserve a similar circuit related to the extended amygdala [my emphasis; McDonald also talks about inhibitory projections to both medial and lateral hypothalamus].

I don't think it's necessary here to discuss the microanatomy of amydgalar complex. A distinction between its corticobasolateral and centromedial subnuclei is serviceable enough. Nor do I find it useful for present purposes to identify all the dozen-or-so bed nuclei to which Dumont alluded at the start of this chapter.

Suffice it to say that we're on the hunt to conceptualize our study of subcortex. So far, we've identified aspects of an interface between telencephalon and diencephalon about which we need more information. See "**Diencephalon**, embryology of."

4.

Claustrum

What is subcortex, aside from an obvious thought about something beneath cortex? Are there general functional aspects of subcortex? Take the case of a cloistered, deep structure, the claustrum (claustrum means "that which is cloistered").

*

Say what you will about hullabaloo caused by Crick and Koch in 2005, but their review of claustrum published that year (Crick died the year before, while writing it) sustains interest if you simply *enjoy* anatomy; a person can almost ignore the argument about claustrum's purported role in consciousness.

Here are some observations summarized by Crick and Koch, with my editorialization based on later papers by others, whom I cite:

1. In horizontal or coronal section, claustrum is a sliver of grey matter deep to the surface of insula with white matter on either side of it (the external and extreme capsules). If visualized as a single, flat surface in the parasagittal plane, it vaguely resembles a map of the contiguous United States. A flattened claustrum, from its east to west coasts, lies within the anterior-posterior extent of the midline *corpus callosum* (Crick and Koch, 2005, reproduced with permission).

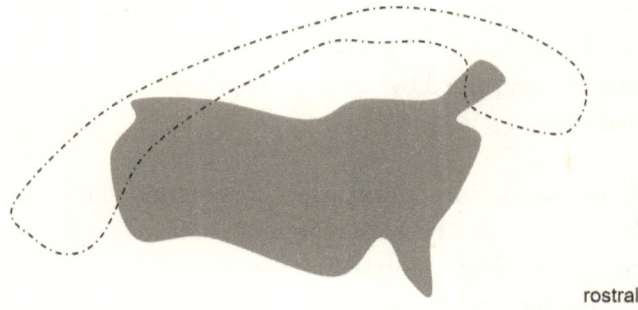
rostral

2. There are relatively few types of neurons in claustrum, compared to the diversity seen elsewhere in cortex. The claustrum's neurons don't form layers. Principal claustral neurons are largely glutamatergic; GABAergic neurons account only for a minority, ~15% (Brown et al., 2017).
3. How the claustrum interconnects with overlying cortex isn't straightforward. Claustrum's east coast projects to (and receives axons from) frontal lobe, but retrograde tracing studies show that frontal locales also project to areas of claustrum from its Atlantic to Pacific coasts. Visual cortex projects to the west coast, but also to points as far east as Colorado, roughly.
4. Per unit cortical volume, claustrum has the highest connectivity with other cortex in the brain; claustral output is basically ipsilateral, but input to it can either be bilateral or preferentially contralateral–the latter specifically in the case of input from motor cortex (Goll et al., 2015).
5. Crick and Koch refer to work (Hadjikhani and Roland, 1998; Roland and Mortensen, 1987) that causes a double-take. Hadjikhani and Roland ask, "how does the brain match visual shape with somatosensory shape? Is it possible that the cortical fields representing visual shape communicate with the cortical fields representing somatosensory shape?"

As Paul Flechsig argued at the very end of the 19th century (discussed in *Frontal Brain and Language*, chapter 5), data from different senses don't communicate in the manner of a handshake (primary area to primary area). Certainly in the newborn, Flechsig observed, "... individual sensory areas are separated from one another by wide tracts of cortex ... in which sensory fibers cannot be followed up." Hadjikhani and Roland don't even allow that multimodal cortical areas are necessarily where matches between, for example, shapes determined by vision and touch transpire. Instead, based on functional imaging:

> We found the insula-claustrum consistently active only when somatosensory shape representations were compared with visual shape representations, whereas we did not find any polymodal areas active during the processing of somatosensory as well as visual shape information.

I won't try to explain—neither do the authors, really—why insula-claustrum on the right in particular, not on both sides, activated. They're content to observe the "claustrum receives and gives rise to direct cortical projections and that it contains maps of different sensory (visual, auditory, and somatosensory) and motor systems."

A person's astonished curiosity can be put in the form of a question: how unimodal is cortex in general; how multimodal is subcortex in general?

6. There's disagreement in the literature (Brown et al., 2017): "recent [claustrum] studies in primate have found little evidence for multimodal responses in passive sensory tasks [yet, Hadjikhani and Roland describe a very active sensory task]. It remains important to determine whether the synaptic organization of the claustrum supports multimodal integration, and whether individual claustral neurons exhibit multimodal responses under specific behavioral conditions."
7. We can't help but note a desire among all authors to comment about what subcortex *does*, at least in some general way.

In the spirit of compare-and-contrast essays from college days, Goll et al. (2015) think about claustrum and thalamus:

> . . . sensory selectivity is one of the most important functions of the brain. Defining what features or objects will be attended, and more importantly (and potentially dangerously) what can be ignored, is crucial for efficient interaction with the surrounding world. Therefore, it

may be beneficial that multiple circuits work to achieve this goal. We propose that both the thalamus and the claustrum have the capacity to focus attention, albeit at different stages of sensory processing.

Simplistically, the different stages are: *early* (in the case of thalamus) and *late* ("late," meaning after some amount of cortical processing, in the case of claustrum).

*

It's all interesting, but our own main business is to continue anatomizing subcortex. And we need to step back before moving forward.

5.

Diencephalon, embryology of

I've discussed this chapter's topic elsewhere (chapters 5 and 7 in *Crossed Organization of Brains*, chapter 3 in *Learning the Brainstem*), but I can't stop trying to depict an important transition in neurodevelopment, well before the end of the first trimester of pregnancy. It's not just that the neural tube closes at roughly gestational day 25 followed by a division into hemispheres roughly after the sixth gestational week. There's also change at the midline and on either side of it.

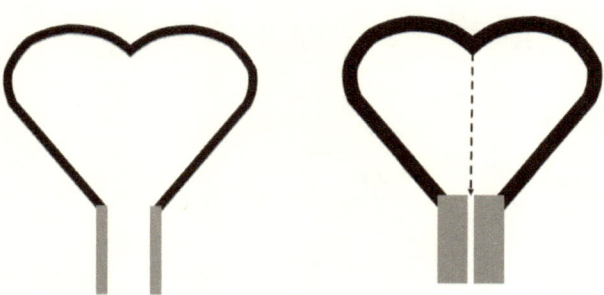

Grey represents developing diencephalon.
Black represents developing telencephalon.
The figure to the right is later than the one on the left.
Dashed line represents the *lamina terminalis*.

The ***lamina terminalis*** becomes the anterior extent or limit of third ventricle, which is the cavity bounded on either side (laterally) by diencephalic structures. Which diencephalic structures?

There's been debate over an answer. Although one source squelches dissent (Nieuwenhuys et al., 2008a), the bones of contention are worth a dust-off and re-examination. Let's start with the apparently unobjectionable:

> During early development, the **ventral thalamus** or *prethalamus* occupies a considerable sector of the wall of the diencephalon. Its matrix zone, which never attains the width of that of **dorsal thalamus**, has been completely depleted by the end of the tenth week. The dorsal and ventral thalami are separated by a cell-free band, the ***zona limitans intrathalamicus*** [for convenience related to what follows, we'll abbreviate this structure as ZLI]. Within this zone, the *lamina medullaris externa* develops. A similar, but less conspicuous limiting zone separates the ventral thalamus from the subthalamus and becomes the *fasciculus thalamicus* [see *"Ansa Lenticularis."* The thalamic fasciculus is also known as Forel field H2]. The column of grey matter between these two limiting zones represents the ventral thalamic premordium, from which the *ventral lateral geniculate nucleus*, the *zona incerta* and the *reticular nucleus* develop.... These nuclei differentiate early; they are already clearly distinguishable in the second half of the third month, during which time the dorsal thalamus is still represented by an undifferentiated primordium [authors' italics].

Enter the controversy:

> The ***subthalamus***, which is characterized by the very early depletion of its ventricular matrix, gives rise to the subthalamic nucleus and, according to [Werner] Kahle and [Paul] Richter, to the internal and external parts of the globus pallidus as well.... During later development the two pallidal primordia were observed to unite with the primordial putamen to form the lentiform nucleus. Recent studies of gene expression patterns [in mice] (particularly that of *Nkx2.1*) have conclusively shown that the globus pallidus derives from an entirely telencephalic primordium.... The interpretation of

the subthalamus as a separate diencephalic entity is not generally accepted. [Hartwig] Kuhlenbeck incorporated the entire subthalamic zone in the hypothalamus and, according to several recent authors who used molecular genetic techniques, the globus pallidus is of telencephalic rather than of diencephalic origin.[4]

The likes of Kahle, Richter, and Kuhlenbeck date to a prior generation of anatomists (I read Kahle as a medical student, so maybe we're talking a couple of generations back). Truth be known, however, molecular biology hasn't demonstrated an irrefutably discrete division between telencephalon and diencephalon (for a relevant discussion, see Trujillo et al., 2005).

I'll borrow from a couple of sources about what can be said without fuss—these two reviews introduce me to a rich-like-cake, addicting literature. In the first, Lim and Golden (2007) straightforwardly say that: (1.) the diencephalon is the embryonic precursor to the caudal forebrain, and that (2.) the major diencephalic structure in the mature animal (a lot of research having been done not only in the chick and mouse, but also in non-vertebrates, like *Drosophila*) is thalamus.[5]

Just those two observations strike me as provocative—in the sense of forcing me to think for myself. If *globus pallidus* is of telencephalic origin, then pallidal-thalamic connectivity is a route by which telencephalon communicates with diencephalon—which seems a tad backward, because we tend to think of thalamus as a way station for ascending input to cortex. Swanson perhaps overreached—not without interesting reasons for

---

[4] Not to get too lost in the weeds, but there's an additional question about the embryology of the ***substantia nigra pars reticulata***, which is an output nucleus as is medial GP. GABA-positive cell populations in the basal plate ventral to the developing diencephalon have been identified in human embryos (Verney et al., 2001); those GABA-positive cells migrate variously throughout a territory that extends from midbrain to subthalamus, but some likely contribute to the mature pars reticulata. In frogs, toads, and mammals like rats, "medial GP" is an "**entopeduncular nucleus**" which is of pallidal origin, but the story in ray-finned fish may differ. In the zebrafish, entopeduncular nucleus arises from "**thalamic eminences**" or *eminentia thalami*, which are not pallidal (Wulliman and Mueller, 2004).

[5] The astute reader is bothered that we don't mention hypothalamus as a major diencephalic structure. I invite her to consult "**Infundibulum**," below.

doing so–in contemplating a **cortico-striatal-pallidal-thalamo-cortical organization** relevant to amygdala (discussed in our chapter three); we've considered the apparently shared function of claustrum and thalamus in information selection relevant to cortical function generally (discussed in our chapter four). Does the border between telencephalon and diencephalon– the two together are "prosencephalon"–relate to information transfer that happens at very least between those two parts of a whole prosencephalon?

For more education about events at the diencephalic-telencephalic border, we have a second review that traces progress from early work in gene expression during development (e.g., Fraser et al., 1990) to more recent wisdom about what any boundary really might be:

> Boundary formation and the activity of local signaling centers are key features of vertebrate brain development. Although a good case has been made for the hindbrain [think: brainstem] forming in a segmented fashion, there is little evidence for a neuromeric organization[6] of the forebrain. In this area, the emerging diencephalic subregions have individual molecular profiles but lack the shared, reiterated features that characterize a segmental ground plan. It is tempting to speculate that the phylogenetically younger forebrain shows greater morphological variability between different species because it is less restricted by compartmental organization (Kiecker and Lumsden, 2005).

"Phylogenetic youth," as could be said of young age in general, enjoys options afforded not only by the liberty of an extended future, but also by all the metamorphoses of a brain starting at an early, gestational age. How information gets to telencephalon, or even from one place to another within telencephalon (think: claustrum), is the issue. One author has discussed the matter of cortical "afferentation" in a general sense–i.e., more than just sensory data finding their way to cortex (Luria, 1973). We've spoken of

---

[6] The authors define "neuromeric organization" for us as "the segmental organization of the neuroepithelium."

information selection—"channeling"[7] of data may be a better term. Is it the upshot of all kinds of developmental metamorphoses?

In the transition from diencephalon to telencephalon, a reiterated ground-plan doesn't serve the kind of work for which the vaunted telencephalon will be responsible in time. Why would complexity diminish in the development towards a mature prosencephalon? (Just as a reminder, "prosencephalon" includes both telencephalon and diencephalon.)

*

Returning to a pregnant thought about "activity of local signaling centers," can we identify just one center? Nieuwenhuys et al. provide an example: the ZLI, they say, is the area where the **external (or lateral) medullary lamina of thalamus** will develop in time. In the adult, that lamina is a myelinated strand of intrathalamic tissue, different from the **internal medullary lamina of thalamus**. The external lamina separates reticular nucleus of thalamus from both dorsal and ventral thalamic nuclei. In development, however, ZLI is a central zone that "signals" what, exactly?

ZLI, also called a **mid-diencephalic organizer**, appears after neural tube closure; it's "the last brain signaling center to form and the first forebrain compartment to be established" (Sena et al., 2016). Anterior to ZLI is prethalamus, also known as ventral thalamus. Posterior to it is thalamus, also known as dorsal thalamus. Note that adjectives like "ventral" and "dorsal" refer, in the embryo, to positions along the anterior-posterior axis, hence the attendant use of "pre" thalamus (in front) as opposed to "thalamus" located more posteriorly along the neural tube. As a compartment that separates rostral/front from caudal/back in the developing diencephalon, ZLI prevents intermingling of anterior and posterior cells and, based on positions *relative to* ZLI, use of signals (e.g., the effects of sonic hedgehog expression) will differ (Kiecker and Lumsden, 2005; Fuccillo et al., 2006). Sena et al. (2016) add that ZLI is "the only part of the dorsal neural tube expressing the morphogen Sonic Hedgehog (Shh) [emphasis on "dorsal," because Shh elsewhere is ventrally concentrated, as in ventral telencephalon] whose activity participates in the

---

[7] I mean "channeling" in the sense of changing channels (maybe volume, too, as in watching TV) rather than of "funneling."

survival, growth, and patterning of neuronal progenitor subpopulations within the thalamic complex."

By drawing attention to how *globus pallidus* must be telencephalic–specifically *not* what Werner Kahle (1986) called a motor zone of diencephalon–, we end up contemplating how early prosencephalic development builds on the ZLI as an organizing, central compartment in diencephalon–and, by a reasonable extension of that line of thought, how telencephalon builds on ZLI as that "first forebrain compartment to be established."

6.

Eminences

I'll discuss two. Both are embryonic structures which protrude into the lateral ventricular cavity. They are the **medial and lateral ganglionic eminences**, **MGE** and **LGE**, respectively:

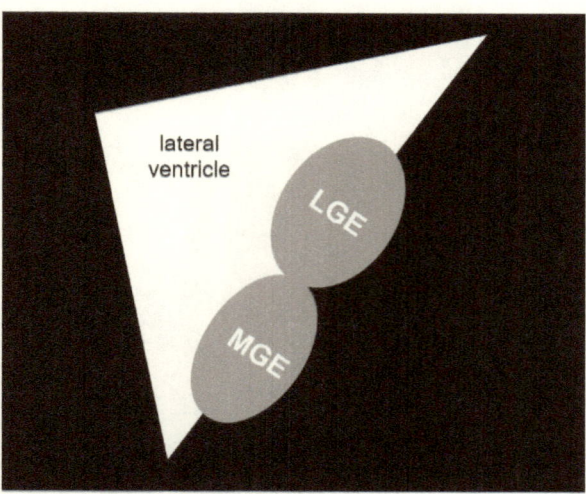

In a way that would give a card-carrying developmental neuroscientist the fits, think about the above schematic in relationship to a hemibrain in coronal section stained for myelin. I'll ask that you basically ignore the internal capsule, which develops late in gestation. Here we view an adult brain, so the internal capsule is present, traversed by one biggish, but incomplete bridge of grey;[8] the white arrow marks a part of anterior commissure:

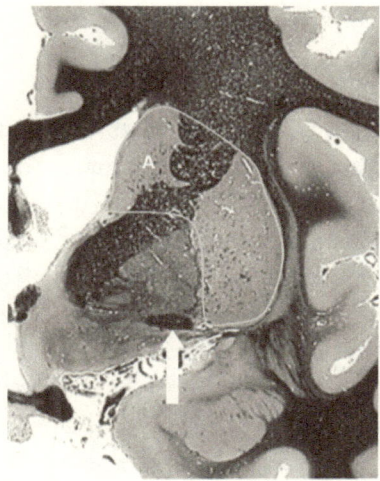

The outline indicates a single domain, marked as "A." What is A's relationship to the embryonic LGE?

Here's the same coronal section, with different domain indicated by a rectangle; we'll name it "B":

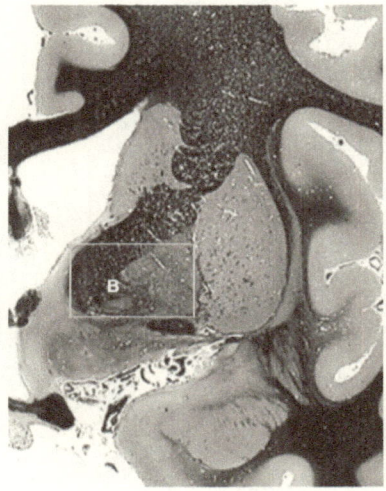

---

[8] The anatomical term for the bridges (which have their own myelin) across the internal capsule is: "Wilson's pencils" (Carpenter and Peter, 1972).

Domain B would reach the ventricular surface medially, were it not for the internal capsule. What is B's relationship to the embryonic MGE?

Traditionally, MGE has been assumed to develop into adult globus pallidus, *and LGE into mature caudate and putamen (or* corpus striatum*).*

Enter complexity:

> ... new developmental data have complicated this scheme [see the italicized sentence, above] due to the existence of: (1) multiple progenitor subdivisions within both LGE and MGE, each giving rise to different neuron subpopulations, a question that is still being investigated, and (2) tangential migration of neurons from MGE and other embryonic domains to the developing striatum, but also from LGE and other embryonic domains to the developing pallidum, contributing to neuronal diversity found in the mature nuclei of the basal ganglia (Medina et al., 2014).

Consider yet another periventricular structure; we're still using the same coronal image:

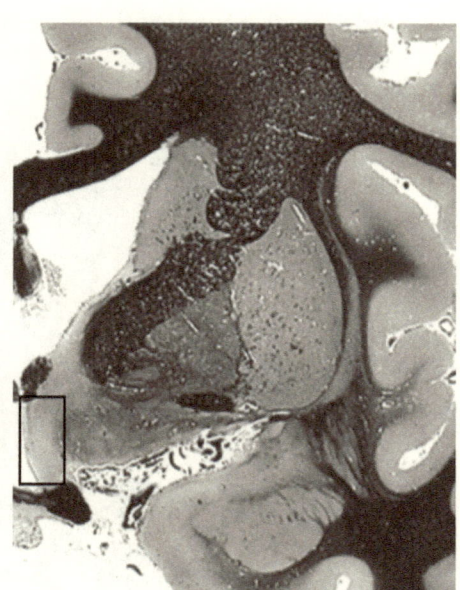

Preoptic Area (POA)

Embryonic **POA,** a progenitor zone just as MGE and LGE are, also generates *globus pallidus* neurons (Nóbrega-Pereira et al., 2010) and even neurons in medial amygdala (Hirata et al., 2009).

*

The science behind radial vs. tangential migration in development is beyond the scope of this chapter and monograph, but three basic points can be made. First, neurons (and non-neurons for that matter) originate in places different from where they are found in the adult brain (Marín and Rubenstein, 2001). Second, the distinction between radial and tangential migration isn't difficult to understand; it can be schematized:

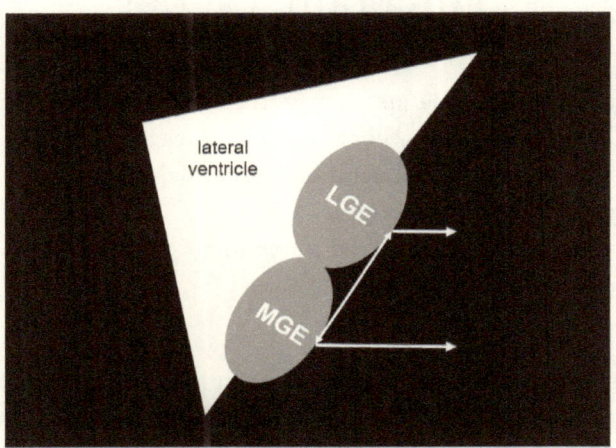

I include only the bidirectional tangent between MGE and LGE. Radial migration from both those progenitor zones—and from others that we haven't discussed—extends outward, perhaps to cortex (two arrows pointing to the right of the image). Third, since our interest has been GABAergic projections from an adult output nucleus (e.g., medial GP or medial amygdala), and although it's not the case that all GABAergic neurons and interneurons arise from the same progenitor zones, we can say in general that subcortical telencephalon produces various GABAergic neurons, including projection neurons (e.g., from *corpus striatum* to *globus pallidus* or *globus pallidus* to thalamus) as well as interneurons which relocate to work in mature isocortex (Anderson et al., 2001).[9]

---

[9] GABAergic neurons account for ~20% of cortical neurons; they provide

7.

Forebrain, caudal

"Caudal forebrain" is a just synonym for diencephalon, but the word "forebrain" has connotations. For one, it connotes telencephalon and all its pyramidal and nonpyramidal neurons; pyramidal neurons, which account for the majority, are glutamatergic.

Is there a glutamatergic caudal forebrain?

*

If we think developmentally, there must be some identifiable process that determines whether a pluripotent cell in a progenitor zone becomes, say, GABAergic, glutamatergic, or something else. In caudal forebrain, such induction depends on at least two things: first the cell must be prepared to receive a signal–the cell must be "competent" to respond; second, there has to be the inducing signal.

In a study of chick embryos (Robertshaw et al., 2013), a thalamic/diencephalic domain immediately adjacent to ZLI (see "**Diencephalon, embryology of**") gives rise to GABAergic neurons, whereas induction of glutamatergic thalamus happens at a distance from ZLI. Molecular specification of how such a "prepattern" emerges has been described in other species; the suggestion, then, is that there's a conserved mechanism,

---

"inhibitory tone to cortical projection (glutamatergic) neurons," according to Anderson et al. Their variety also has to do with differing neuropeptide content in any given GABAergic neuronal pool.

at least among amniotes like birds and mammals. So, sure, there's both a GABAergic and glutamatergic caudal forebrain.

But the question, asked at the start of this chapter and just answered preliminarily, is a loaded one.

*

Alert. A digression follows.

Let's say that you've been teaching at a medical school for about 30 years, starting in an era before the PDF. So, early on, you collected actual books, many of which went untouched after purchase perhaps, but you had a sense that they were worth the money. Over years, you consulted them occasionally, but a good number—you admitted it to yourself—were out of your intellectual league. Then, you happen to be writing something one day, and you recall a chapter in a book still on the shelf. You're now interested to see what became of the information in the chapter. Let's look at Sherman (2017) writing about thalamus roughly 20 years after first exposure to him. The book off the aforementioned shelf (mine), in case you're curious, is *The Synaptic Organization of the Brain* in its fourth edition, published in 1998.

Sherman launches a shot across the bow of a traditional view of thalamus:

> That view goes something like this. Information from the periphery is relayed in a rather machine-like manner through certain thalamic nuclei to cortex. That information is then processed entirely within cortex via various intracortical pathways until executive areas are reached, from which outputs to brainstem or spinal sites are sent to affect behavior. This sensorimotor processing that occurs within cortex has no significant thalamic involvement, and thus the role of thalamus is limited to relaying peripheral information to cortex. In other words, except for the few thalamic nuclei that relay peripheral information to cortex, the rest of thalamus, which is the large majority by volume, has little to do (Sherman, 2017).

I love the first sentence, which drips with irony of course. He's not about to defend the view, nor did he 20 years before:

> . . . the thalamus does much more than merely act as a passive and machine-like relay of information to cortex. Instead, the ability to pass through this gateway is determined by specialized neuronal circuitry: the gate can be completely open, which results in the relay of all information to cortex; completely closed, which cuts off cortex from the outside world; or partially open, which permits certain information to reach cortical levels. Also, the special properties of relay cells can strongly influence the nature of the thalamic relay (Sherman and Koch, 1998).

Thalamic relay cells, which are excitatory, project to all layers of cortex (Douglas and Martin, 2010). The excitation–the "drive" afforded by the thalamocortical projection–can be weak (Bruno and Sakmann, 2010) until, perhaps, the aperture of the gate changes. The gate is bidirectional. "Numerically impressive" glutamatergic, corticothalamic projections input to all known thalamic cell types (McCormick, 2010).

8.

Globus Pallidus, lateral (in particular)

A useful strategy for a teacher is to rethink what she has taught from time to time. Some statements seem–emphasis on "seem"–to survive with their truth value intact. For example:

> *Medial* globus pallidal *neurons physiologically behave like those of the* substantia nigra pars reticulata.
>
> *So, the* pars reticulata *is an output nucleus as is the medial* globus pallidus. (See "**Diencephalon**, embryology of.")

Or:

> *The structures of the* **corpus striatum**, *including the* **caudate**, **putamen**, nucleus accumbens septi, *and olfactory tubercle, arise from the same embryonic rest of tissue.* (See "**Nucleus accumbens septi**" and "**Olfactory tubercle**.")

Or:

> *Dopaminergic projections from the* **substantia nigra pars compacta** *project to the* corpus striatum (See "**Olfactory tubercle**.")

Others might need tweaking sooner rather than later. For example:

> *Lateral* globus pallidus *(abbreviated in a moment as* "GPe"*) projects to subthalamic nucleus of Luys* (STN) *in the* **indirect pathway**.

It's not that any of the statements is clearly wrong, but do they need pedagogical overhaul? Perhaps they all do, but I want to concentrate on the last of them in this chapter.

*

Here's a summary of a heuristic scheme used to teach about the basal ganglia:

> An important model of basal ganglia dysfunction, commonly used to explain the motor symptoms of Parkinson's disease (PD), implies that the interaction of the STN and GPe is unidirectional and constant over time. It also accounts for the symptoms of PD in terms of changes in the mean rates of activity of basal ganglia nuclei. Thus, abnormal over-activity of the GABAergic neurons projecting from the striatum to the GPe reduces the activity of the GPe, which results in disinhibition of the STN and, in turn, drives over-activity of the basal ganglia output nuclei and excessive inhibition of their targets. In contrast to the proposed pathological over-activity of this 'indirect pathway' to the output nuclei, the 'direct pathway' (i.e., the direct projection from the striatum [to medial globus pallidus]) is proposed to be relatively under-active. Therefore, the reduced inhibition of basal ganglia output nuclei also contributes to their relative over-activity in PD (Bevan et al., 2002).

The five sentences elaborate on a cortico-striatal-pallidal-thalamo-cortical organization that we've discussed elsewhere in this book. A keen eye might focus on two words and one phrase in the passage: *unidirectional*; *constant*; and *mean rates of activity*.

*

Unidirectionality. Wilson (1998) tells us that there are approximately 111 million neurons in the human **neostriatum** (bilateral caudates plus putamens). Roughly half that number projects to lateral *globus pallidus* ("lateral GP" henceforward). Hardman et al. (2002) studied five human brains without neuropsychiatric disease either clinically or neuropathologically (three women, two men; mean age 74 years); they counted neurons in lateral GPs to give us a rough number of 1.45 million per brain. A unidirectional projection from neostriatum to lateral GPs would thus be associated with an convergence ratio of ~100 to 1.

Some argue (Bevan et al., 2002) that there's a return projection from lateral GP to neostriatum, and there's divergence to match the convergence in the opposite direction. But there may be differences in the synaptic connections made in either destination.

Regarding how many STN neurons there are in a human brain, the answer is ~561,000 (Hardman et al., 2002), so there's a convergence ratio from lateral GP to STN of ~2.6 to 1. Working in the opposite direction, from STN to lateral GP, the divergence is the inverse, with the same qualification regarding terminal arbors and other synaptic considerations on either side.

Convergence is what people think about when they unidirectionally, but, as in the case of bidirectional striatonigral and nigrostriatal projections (Bevan et al., 2002 and Crittenden et al., 2016), we should probably reflect on the *back and forth* that characterize key connections *before* any projection to output nuclei, whether medial GP or the *pars reticulata* of *substantia nigra*.

*

Constancy. Even in a limited experience with (aural) microelectrode monitoring during functional neurosurgery targeting deep structures, it's hard not to notice that there's a difference in how neostriatum *sounds* as opposed to, say, STN in a parkinsonian patient. Striatum is quiet; STN is consistently loud.

Bolam (2010) offers two reasons for the difference, whether in the disease state (as in Parkinson's disease) or in a normal brain. Under resting conditions, medium spiny neurons of the neostriatum are relatively hyperpolarized and thus quiescent. Also, when excitatory/glutamatergic input does happen–input comes from either cortex or thalamus–the response of medium spiny neurons depends on local collaterals of those spiny neurons and the activity of GABAergic interneurons in that collateral circuitry. Beven et al. (2002) add that, by comparison, neurons of the STN and lateral GP spontaneously and rhythmically fire even when they are disconnected from input. Even in the normal state, they are noisy. Likewise, output nuclei, including medial GP and *pars reticulata* of the *substantia nigra*, are tonically active in the normal brain (Bolam, 2010).

So, corticostriatal or thalamostriatal input isn't constant, and bidirectional wiring between lateral GP and STN contributes to the tonic activity of both lateral GP and STN. But there's more to the story.

*

Mean rates of activity. Together, pattern and rate of an input, as opposed to its mean firing rate, can result in interesting and counterintuitive effects. If, as we just read, lateral GP neurons fire rhythmically as do STN neurons, but not necessarily at the same rhythm and not necessarily as a consequence of cortical or striatal discharge beforehand, then what net effect can one predict from GABAergic output from lateral GP?

As it happens, the pattern and rate of an inhibitory input from lateral GP determines not just the inhibition of STN, but also and perhaps more importantly whether STN neurons will fire in spikes or bursts. Inhibitory input from lateral GP can "contribute to the range of firing patterns expressed by STN neurons *in vivo*." What's more, "firing mode of STN neurons is related more intimately to the magnitude *and pattern* of inhibitory input than to the frequency of input averaged over long periods . . . [and] *can actually augment, rather than reduce*, the activity of STN neurons (my italics, Bevan et al., 2002).

*

So, yes, absolutely: lateral GP projects to STN in the indirect pathway.

It's a statement that opens a wormhole as described in physics, a passageway in theory to unexpected places or knowledge. I rather believe that wormholes exist for those who study the brain.

9.

Habenula

I have a specific reason to discuss it (mainly having to do with dopamine), but, first, where is it in a human brain?

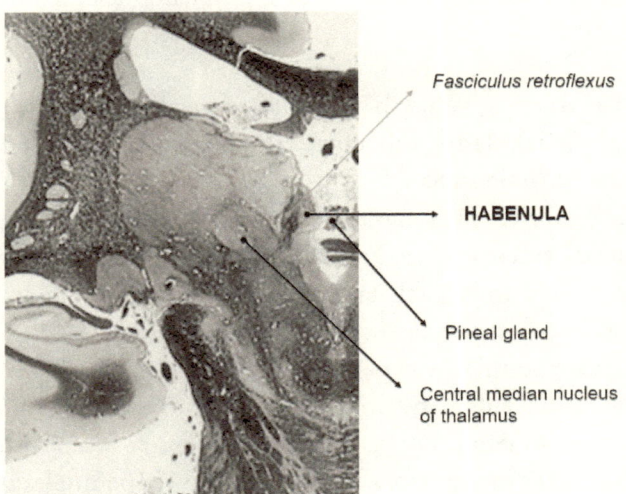

The above coronal section, which stains white matter black, is at the level of the posterior commissure. In the rhesus monkey, in a coronal section stained for cells, one can visualize two parts of habenula; the medial habenula stains more darkly:

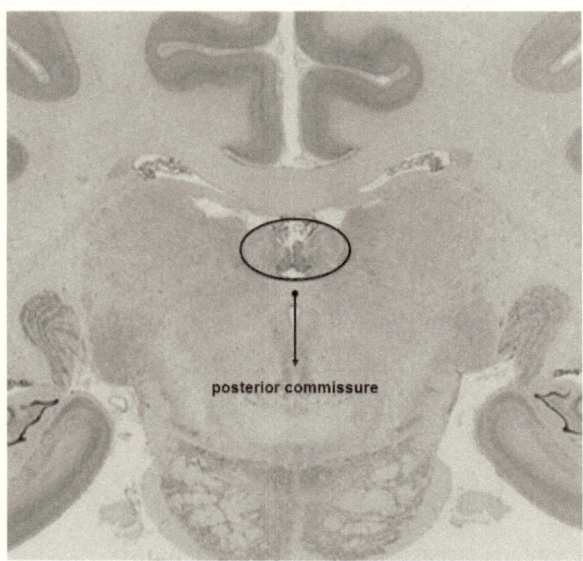

Now let's consider five observations, all anatomical, about habenula (Hikosaka, 2010):

1. It's a structure found in almost all vertebrate species.
2. The **pineal gland**, habenula, and ***stria medullaris thalami*** derive from **epithalamus**.
3. Habenula receives input from limbic system and neostriatum (**dorsal striatum**) mainly through the *stria medullaris thalami*, which is plainly visible on the medial surface of human thalamus.
4. Habenular output passes via the *fasciculus retroflexus*, also known as the **habenula-interpeduncular tract**.
5. Lateral habenular neurons project, via *fasciculus retroflexus*, both to dopaminergic nuclei (*substantia nigra pars compacta* and the **ventral tegmental area of Tsai**) and to **raphe nuclei** involved in indolamine neurotransmission.

With bravura and intelligence, Hikosaka (2010) hypothesizes that "first, the role of the habenula is to suppress motor activity; and second, the habenula is activated under adverse conditions." He elaborates, with reference to **lateral and medial divisions of habenula (LHb** and **MHb**, respectively):

The motor suppression that is associated with aversion prediction may be mediated by the LHb-dopamine circuit—because the majority of LHb neurons are excited by aversive events— leading to an inhibition of dopamine neurons that consequently leads to a general suppression of body movements. In addition, the aversion predicting activation of the LHb (and possibly the MHb) activates serotonin neurons in the raphe nuclei and therefore influences neural processing in a large part of the brain, although the specific behavioural outcomes of LHb-mediated serotonin modulations are still unclear.

Inhibition and excitation are nuanced rather than obligate actions, variable in magnitude and temporal pattern. The baseline states of putatively inhibitory or excitatory centers figure into whether those centers actually inhibit or excite others.

The influence of a diffusely projecting system (e.g., dopamine) on telencephalon is a function of such subcortical channeling–of information, of excitation and inhibition. We have accumulated a number of examples of channeling:

>medial GP to thalamus ("inhibitory"); see *"Ansa lenticularis"*;
>thalamus to cortex ("excitatory"); see "**Forebrain**, caudal";
>extended amygdala to thalamus/hypothalamus ("inhibitory");
>see "**Bed nuclei of the *Stria Terminalis***";
>claustrum to cortex ("excitatory"); see "**Claustrum**";
>lateral GP/STN network to medial GP ("inhibitory");
>see *"Globus Pallidus*, lateral (in particular)";
>lateral habenula to dopaminergic nuclei ("inhibitory");
>discussed in the present chapter.

"Inhibitory" and "excitatory," in each case, refers to the main neurotransmitter used in the projection, but the net effect of the output depends on contexts that vary in time.

10.

Infundibulum

Wilhelm His, Sr. (1831-1904) identified infundibulum at the tip of the early neural plate in chordate and vertebrate species. In a "fate map" based on three-week-old shark embryos, he envisioned that the pituitary gland would develop in a location caudal to both the oropharyngeal membrane and to the neural plate's leading edge, the *lamina terminalis* (Swanson, 2012b). Infundibulum is continuous posteriorly with a bulge in the floor of the third ventricle, the ***tuber cinereum***.

Hypothalamus *is* a diencephalic structure, but its proximity to rostral telencephalic structures, including basal forebrain nuclei, introduces problems for those who try to identify specific, gene-based prosomeric boundaries in development. Some have gone so far as to refer to a "secondary" prosencephalon (telencephalon plus hypothalamus) that exhibits "patterning singularities" different from the developing diencephalon (Puelles and Rubenstein, 2003). One peculiarity we might notice in light of our talk about lateral GP and STN (see "***Globus pallidus, lateral*** [in particular]") is the fate map of a structure like STN, whose cells have long been thought to arise in the floor of developing hypothalamus (Gilbert, 1935 and Marchand, 1987).

I'm not about to discuss hypothalamic anatomy with any gruesome rigor. But if we use infundibulum as a landmark, we can start to understand hypothalamus and its bidirectional relationship to cortex.

Let's begin at the level of the optic chiasm in a coronal section stained for cells, not white matter:

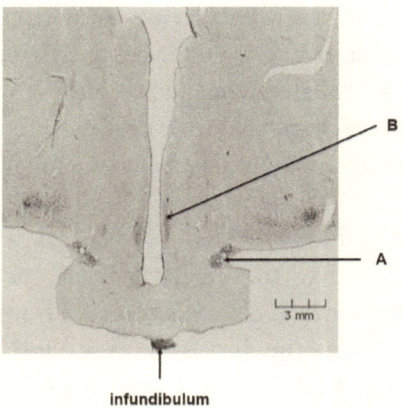

infundibulum

Two cell groups marked A and B just on one side of the image are **supraoptic** and **paraventricular** nucleus, respectively.[10] The unmarked, laterally located clusters of cells are **basal nuclei of Meynert** in the basal forebrain (see "**Quadrilateral Space of Broca**").

Magnocellular components of both supraoptic and paraventricular nuclei include vasopressin and oxytocin cells that project to posterior pituitary (Harris and Loewy, 1990). Paraventricular nucleus can be divided into other subparts, one of which gives rise to autonomic efferents that pass to brainstem and cord (Luiten et al., 1985).

Still using infundibulum as a (now-virtual) landmark, further caudally towards the tuber cinereum, the cellular aggregates change; their borders are less distinct:

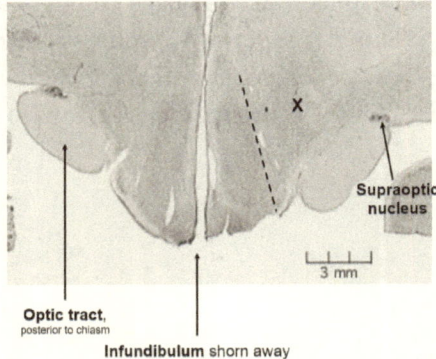

Optic tract, posterior to chiasm

Infundibulum shorn away

---

[10] Another structure of interest is the **suprachiasmatic nucleus**, which isn't visible in this section. It sits atop chiasm *anterior to* the level of infundibulum.

The dashed line marks what seems a division between a medial cellular collection (most, but not all of it being the **ventromedial nucleus of hypothalamus**[11]) and a lateral area, where the "X" is placed, just on one side of the image. **Lateral hypothalamic area** extends further caudally, but we'll pause here to digest a summary about its significance:

> The picture that emerges for descending cortical projections is that the major output for autonomic control by the cerebral cortex is directed from the medial prefrontal cortex, the insular cortex, and the central nucleus of amygdala to the lateral hypothalamus. . . . Descending cortical projections to regions in the medial part of the hypothalamus, controlling endocrine responses, come from the medial nucleus of the amygdala and the hippocampal formation, particularly the subiculum. Finally, cortical projections that are likely to mediate behavioral responses come from the prefrontal cortex, the lateral and basal amygdaloid nuclei, and the hippocampal formation to both the lateral hypothalamus and to the medial nuclei (Saper, 2000).

In terms of hypothalamic projections *to* cortex, we can concentrate on tuberal lateral hypothalamus (with orexin-hypocretin as an important neurotransmitter). It projects topographically: the more lateral in the lateral hypothalamic area, the more lateral the projection throughout the ipsilateral cerebral hemisphere, front to back throughout the hemisphere. Those projections have to do, Saper says, with both feeding and arousal.

There's more to say as we wander posteriorly towards mammillary bodies in hypothalamus. See "**Juxtallocortical Connection (to Hypothalamus)**."

---

[11] If one cares to know more about dorsal-ventral midline nuclei at this level, one can think *in relationship* to ventromedial nucleus: **dorsomedial nucleus** is dorsal to it; **arcuate nucleus** is ventral to it, just above where the infundibulum should be.

11.

Juxtallocortical Connection (to Hypothalamus)

Juxtallocortex and its synonyms **periallocortex** and **mesocortex** refer to structures *close to* allocortex. For "allo-" or "other" cortex, read: paleocortex (rhinencephalon) and archicortex (hippocampus). There are histological reasons to distinguish juxtallocortex from neocortex (for a discussion, see Braak et al., 2000), but I want to think about the juxtallocortical limbic projection to hypothalamus via **fornix** to **mammillary body**, simply because it's a connection that all of us learn in early neuroscience.

Frequently these days, despite ongoing currency of the concept in our teaching, experts cite a problem with James Papez's circuit:

> The role of the hippocampal projection to the hypothalamus remains remarkably enigmatic. Although it was proposed by Papez in 1937 as one leg of a 'circuit' for reverberating emotional sensation, each of the sites in the circuitous pathway that Papez proposed (i.e., the hippocampus to the mammillary body; to the anterior thalamic nuclei; to the cingulate cortex; and back to the hippocampus) contains multiple subdivisions with complex connectivity. There is no credible evidence for circuitous transfer of information in these pathways or for reverberation (Saper, 2000).

I've maintained elsewhere (chapter two in *Teaching Hippocampal Anatomy*) that Papez's interest in a "medial wall" of brain–with hippocampus and hypothalamus at the center of that construct–is the real interest for our century, not his circuit. Advocates of a "greater limbic system" say much the same thing; they'd broaden the "medial" of Papez's medial wall to include much of the neuraxial midline: "The central limbic continuum does not end at the caudal diencephalic or mesencephalic levels, but rather extends throughout the brain stem (Nieuwenhuys et al., 2008e)."

*

It's been rightly observed that fornical fibers don't all terminate in mammillary body; perhaps not even the majority reach there. Alternative termini include thalamus, septal nuclei, ventromedial and lateral nuclei of hypothalamus (we drew attention to the latter two in "**Infundibulum**").

In posterior hypothalamic sections in any atlas, the myelinated fornix and **mammillothalamic tract (of Vicq d'Azyr)** are hard to miss. Myelination can mean different things: microscopic myelin at 400x is still (perhaps "early") myelin, but it's not an "electric blue" (presumably mature) myelin visible to the naked eye in H&E-Luxol Fast Blue slides (Kinney et al., 1988). Posterior hypothalamus has its share of very myelinated tracts *within* hypothalamus, if visualize with the right staining technique:

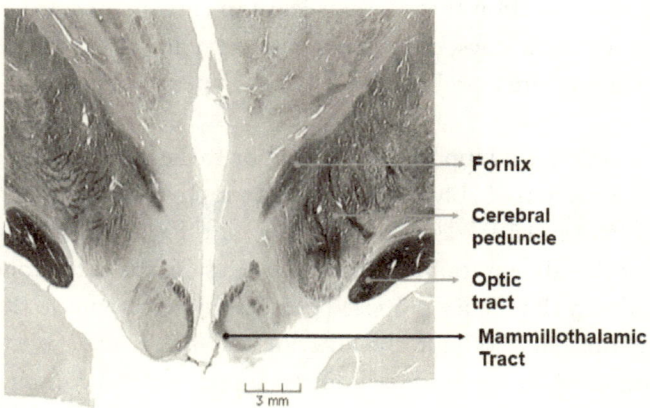

→ Fornix

→ Cerebral peduncle

→ Optic tract

→ Mammillothalamic Tract

3 mm

I wonder why myelin both to and from mammillary bodies is so visible; perhaps the fiber density of fornix and mammillothalamic tract contributes to the visual effect.[12] But given hypothalamic interconnectivity in general at all its levels (cortical projections to and from; septal, brainstem, and juxtallocortical projections to and from), couldn't one envision myelin everywhere in hypothalamus, to some degree?

*

Posterior hypothalamic nuclei that we visualize (more or less) with the help of a cell stain relate to others that we've discussed:

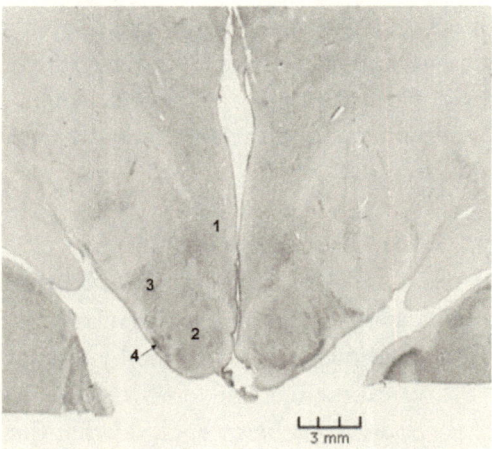

"1" marks the area of **posterior hypothalamus**, which arises from the lateral hypothalamic area noted in the last chapter. "2" marks a **medial mammillary nucleus**, to be distinguished from a **lateral mammillary nucleus** ("3"). The separation between them has, in part, to do with the appearance of both fornix and mamillothalamic tract in gestation. "4" marks a collection of histaminergic cells responsible for histaminergic

---

[12] In an interview available on YouTube (https://youtu.be/mX–k6_n5is), Walle Nauta describes how fine the individual fibers of fornix are. His silver method, which took years to realize, was an attempt better to visualize degenerating fibers specifically in hypothalamus. The Nauta method had wide application in neuroscience before the advent of other retrograde tracing methodologies (see **"Labeled Line"**).

innervation of bilateral cerebral cortex (**tuberomammillary nucleus**; it receives significant input from limbic forebrain [Ericson et al., 1991]).

*

Here are helpful observations from a study of gestational hypothalamus in humans (Koutcherov et al., 2003):

> The earliest observable structural differentiation of the hypothalamus involves the lateral hypothalamic zone, which gives rise to the lateral hypothalamic area, posterior hypothalamus, and lateral tuberal nucleus [the last not to be confused with tuberomammillary nucleus].... [T]he lateral hypothalamic zone relates, broadly speaking, to arousal and feeding.
>
> A second wave of neurogenesis involves nuclei of a hypothalamic "core" characterized by limbic afferents from the amygdala and septum and major intrahypothalamic connections. Two major nuclei of the hypothalamic core include the ventromedial and dorsomedial nuclei and mammillary body. Koutcherov et al. say that the core has fundamentally to do with autonomic responses and to the regulation of homeostasis.
>
> The last to be generated are the neurons considered critical for the regulation of biological rhythms, neuroendocrine output, and integrated autonomic responses, including suprachiasmatic, paraventricular, supraoptic, and arcuate nuclei.

What time frame do we discuss? Hypothalamus develops starting from an early period (certainly by the ninth or tenth gestational week), then until the 34th gestational week (rather late, wouldn't you say?), after which it resembles adult hypothalamus.

12.

Kern

. . . is the German word for both "kernel" and, in an anatomical context, "nucleus."

I like the monosyllabic simplicity and the association with something seedlike or concentrated.

Cajal drew attention to the condensation of tissue in brains that allows for efficient operation (Swanson, 2012a). He spoke of the centralization of function that's a key to neural architecture.

My thoughts about nuclei are informed by Cajalian centralization and a question Pasko Rakic asked 25 years ago. Rakic contemplated differences in cortical surface area between rats, macaque monkeys, and humans. Approximate ratios between the three would be 1 to 100 to 1,000. Then he wondered why, over the 20-odd million years since the macaque and human diverged from some common ancestor, the cortex has seen different rates of expansion in surface area without much of a change in cortical thickness. "What is the explanation," he wrote, "for the approximately 15-fold larger number of postmitotic cells becoming distributed in the form of a thin, regular sheet rather than in a lump or globe, as has occurred during enlargement of the neostriatum [or pallidum or thalamus] over the same evolutionary period?" (Rakic, 1995).

For a person interested in subcortex, the words "lump" and "globe" catch the eye. A question naturally arises about the degree to which such nuclei proportionately enlarge across species.

*

In a study that we used earlier in this monograph, Hardman et al. (2002) compared rat, macaque, other monkey, and human brains (see "*Globus Pallidus*, **lateral**, in particular"). As the reader recalls, the study involved cell counts in structures like lateral GP. From rat to macaque to human, the volume of that subcortical nucleus increases. An important next step is to think about proportionality, either in terms of size or cell counts.

Across species, all had relatively similar proportional volumes for the structures examined, including lateral and medial GP, STN, and both parts of the *substantia nigra* (*pars compacta* plus *pars reticulata*). In terms of cell counts, humans had proportionally more internal relay basal ganglionic neurons (STN and lateral GP neurons), even though volumes remained roughly proportional. The study didn't examine neostriatal structures (we'll address them in a moment), but a first comment to make is that the orders-of-magnitude increase in cortical surface area that Rakic mentions isn't associated with *proportional* enlargements of subcortical nuclei across species.

Using a very different methodology concentrating only on volume, Yin et al. (2009) report that across three populations (rhesus and cynomolgus monkeys and humans), monkeys have a larger putamen and caudate nucleus, compared with total brain volume, when matched against humans. In the rat, Oorschot (1996) reported ~2.8 million striatal neurons in a hemibrain, compared to an estimated 100 million striatal neurons total in a whole brain in humans.

The 100 million estimate comes from older work (Lange et al., 1976) that quantified both larger and smaller striatal neurons in normal brains compared to Huntingtonian brains: larger:smaller ratios were 1:175 in the normal group and 1:40 in Huntingtonians. Earlier in this monograph, we used an estimate of 111 million neostriatal neurons–that's Wilson's guess, about a decade after Lange et al. (1998). Yin et al. as well as Hardman et al. refer us to an old-but-still-good study by Harman (not Hardman) and Carpenter (1950), in which volumetric determination across eight primate species including humans found that caudate volume proportionately decreases "as the primate scale is ascended" along with an increase in putaminal volume. But, in the aggregate, we're still not talking about a meaningful difference between humans and primates in terms of neostriatal nuclear volume or cell count in proportion to total brain mass.

*

So, cortical surface area increases by two or more orders of magnitude, but cortical thickness doesn't much change at all, comparatively. And cortical surface area increases but striatal structures proportionate to brain mass don't, even though they do enlarge and their cell counts do increase. A take-home point could be that subcortex connects to or otherwise contends with more cortical surface per unit striatal volume or even per striatal neuron. A contrary view might hold that the cortex does more brain work in humans with less dependency on subcortex.

The latter argument doesn't tally with Cajal's thought about efficiency. In general, he thought that brains exist in the first place because there's biological need for a concentration of resources and the centralization of function.

Cortical elaboration in evolution doesn't obviate nuclei.

13.

Labeled Line

The concept of a labeled line has self-evident utility, up to a point. Here's a perspective from sensory physiologists regarding the phenomenon of taste:

> A labeled line, in the strict sense, means that there is a separate and distinct population of receptor cells for each of the taste qualities (e.g., a population of sweet-sensing taste receptor cells and a separate population of bitter-sensing cells). Moreover, each receptor cell excites dedicated primary afferent fibers that transmit the same signal to the central nervous system (CNS). That is, the afferent fiber becomes a line that is exclusively dedicated to that singular taste quality. Within the CNS, relay and projection neurons for these signals, according to labeled line coding, retain the same label (e.g., "sweet"). Hence, the entire line is uniquely labeled for each taste quality.
>
> There is little experimental evidence for such a strict labeled line in mammalian taste (Roper and Chaudhari, 2018).

So why discuss the concept?

Its self-evident aspect has to do with how one naturally tries to understand any system (not just taste) based on aspects of the experience to which that system is dedicated. A labeled line, say, for color vision is credible, based on the specificity of cones in the retina to detect color, of parvocellular layers in lateral geniculate nucleus to process color after whatever happens in retina, and because there's the anatomical discreteness of cortical color domains (so-called "blobs" in primary visual cortex or V1 and "interstripes" in V2) that receive thalamic or cortical input, respectively.

Enter a competing concept, for which there is much support, according to Roper and Chaudhari:

> In contrast to labeled line coding, combinatorial coding implies that at some point in the pathway, signals in two or more neurons are combined and compared such that the final output represents coactivation of multiple inputs. Consequently, in combinatorial coding, taste qualities (e.g., sweetness) are constructed from a mosaic of activated fibers, none of which conveys all the information needed to distinguish the stimulus if taken alone.

I recall someone who, when eating a sour slice of pineapple, *salted it*. "Makes it sweeter," he said. But prior to the perception of new sweetness of that slice, were there activated, labeled lines for sourness and saltiness that eventually mix in the magic of combinatorial coding? As it happens, as I also learn from the sensory physiologists quoted, a taste bud sensory cell expresses receptors for single qualities. There can be narrow tuning for different tastes.

*

When we apply a labeling concept to lines that pass through basal ganglia and thalamus, it's surprising that parallelism seems the rule more than combination. Here let me review work that I have followed for some years, by a constellation of authors, but the central star for me has been Peter Strick from upstate New York. A problem that he and his colleagues encountered from the late 1970's until the mid-1980's had to do with an inability to follow multisynaptic connections using then-available anatomical techniques. After the advent of viruses as transneuronal tracers, one could follow a line across as many as three synapses.

But let's start in 1979.

An earlier methodology, before viruses, used retrograde tracers such as wheat germ agglutinin conjugated to horseradish peroxidase (WGA-HRP). Two *Macaca* species were studied (Muakkassa and Strick, 1979). To illustrate what they found, I'll use a *Macaca mulatta* brain:

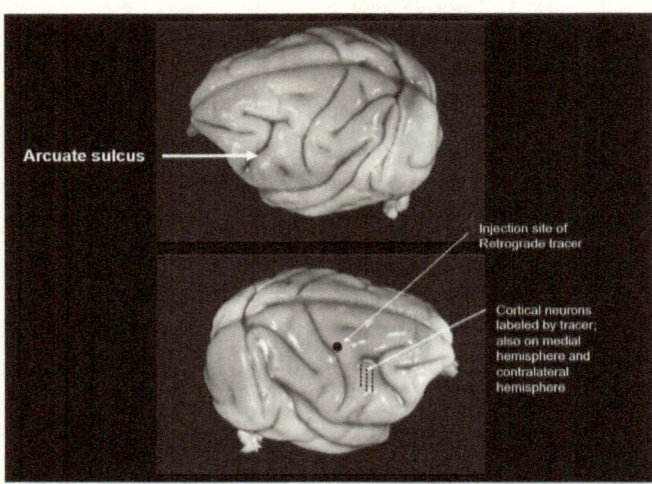

Injection into the arm area of **primary motor cortex** led not only to retrograde labeling primarily in the **arcuate premotor area**, as the image illustrates, but also to **supplementary motor area** on the medial surface of the hemibrain, as well as to the contralateral brain (specifically to arcuate premotor area and supplementary motor area on that other side).

A second injection site was supplementary motor area located medially in a hemibrain (Strick, 1985). The most extensive labeling ensued in a ventrolateral thalamic nucleus; the specific subdivision was the *nucleus ventralis lateralis pars oralis*, in the Olszewski nomenclature for the monkey brain.

A third injection site was the arcuate premotor area. The most extensive labeling happened in a thalamic subdivision that Olszewski mysteriously called "**area X**," which is entirely medial to the area of labeling after injection of supplementary motor area.

Using retrograde tracing with both horseradish peroxidase itself and WGA-HRP, now with initial injections in cervical spinal cord, Dum and Strick (1991) found that primary motor cortex (its arm area) . . . and no less than six premotor areas . . . project to spinal cord. Of the seven *total* premotor-motor areas, we can concentrate on primary motor cortex, arcuate premotor area, and supplementary motor area. It's not just that arcuate premotor and supplementary motor areas themselves project to primary motor cortex, as Muakkassa and Strick learned a few years earlier. In addition,

> . . . like the primary motor cortex, each premotor area has direct access to the spinal cord. Indeed, our findings indicate that the corticospinal system from the premotor areas is numerically as substantial as that from the primary motor cortex.

The authors, interestingly, proceed to specify what *not* to conclude from their findings:

> . . . we do not mean to imply that the premotor areas influence the control of movement only via their corticospinal projections; nor do we mean to imply that the premotor areas function only in parallel with the primary motor cortex. The direct connections of the premotor areas with the primary motor cortex and their participation in cerebellar and basal ganglia loops have long been thought to provide the anatomical substrate for serial interactions between the premotor areas and the primary motor cortex. Instead, we wish to emphasize a viewpoint that has been somewhat neglected, namely, that the premotor areas have parallel outputs directly to the spinal cord that may be independent of these serial interactions (Dum and Strick, 1991).

For "serial interactions," we can be specific, based on our look at work from 1979:

> arcuate premotor area and supplementary motor area **TO** primary motor cortex;
> "area X" **TO** arcuate premotor area; and

nucleus ventralis pars oralis **TO** supplementary motor area.

For "parallel outputs," we have:

primary motor cortex **TO** cord;
"area X" **TO** arcuate premotor area **TO** cord; and
nucleus ventralis pars oralis **TO** supplementary motor area **TO** cord.

*

With the advent of viral methods as used by Strick's group (the viral methods still trace in retrograde fashion), more parallelism emerges, not just with respect to frontal "pre-motor-motor" projections to cord. In this next passage "ventral premotor area" in the *Cebus* monkey is similar to "arcuate premotor area" in *Macaca mulatta* :

> Injections of the McIntyre-B of HSV 1 were made into primary motor area (M1), supplementary motor area (SMA), ventral premotor area (PMv), and frontal eye field (FEF). We found that each of these cortical areas is the target of basal ganglia output. Importantly, the regions of GPi [medial *globus pallidus*] and SNpr [the *pars reticulata* of *substantia nigra*] that were labeled after injections into the different motor areas were separate from each other and from regions labeled after injections into . . . nonmotor areas [e.g., dorsolateral prefrontal cortex *inter alia*] . . . .. Thus, the basal ganglia-thalamocortical system is characterized by multiple parallel pathways to motor and nonmotor areas of the cerebral cortex (Middleton and Strick, 2000).

If we pull one of the original reports summarized in the passage (e.g., Hoover and Strick, 1993), we read that M1, SMA, and PMv injections resulted in retrograde labeling of separate regions of medial GP.

An anatomical specificity of projections wasn't lost upon very early investigators, who used a version of "lesion-the-cortex-then-follow-the-degeneration." In the 1970's, the corticostriatal projection, though observed in cats and other mammals, hadn't been convincingly demonstrated in monkeys. Then investigators like Kemp and Powell observed how non-randomly cortex projects to striatum in primates:

> One of the principal reasons for extending the study of the cortical projection upon the striatum to the monkey brain was to determine whether there was a relationship between the organization of the afferents to the caudate nucleus and putamen on the one hand and the efferents of the external and internal segments of the globus pallidus on the other. It has been shown that the caudate nucleus and putamen project upon the globus pallidus in a well-ordered, topographic manner . . . (Kemp and Powell, 1970).

And, in turn (two decades later), viral transneuronal retrograde tracings identified discrete pallidal territories which project to specific cortical areas. The concept of functionally segregated circuits linking cortex and subcortex back to cortex-of-origin had been advanced years before Strick's results during the 1990's, but reading him in general, for me, makes it hard to ignore the utility of a labeled line concept.
See "**Macro-, Microcircuitry.**"

14.

Macro-, Microcircuitry

Lines begin and end in specific places (see "**Labeled Line**"). With that simple statement in mind, indulge an analogy. The task is to get from home to work, then back home. "Microcircuitry" relates to the various turns taken to accomplish the trip. Routes depend on conditions: weather in particular, and always in a Boston winter, is an X-factor. With the trip in mind, we can organize our thinking about microcircuitry at a macro-level, with focus on the neostriatum (caudate-putamen).

*

<u>Starting from home</u>. We know that principal afferents to the striatum are glutamatergic. They arise both from cortex and thalamus, but we'll concentrate on those from cortex. The afferents synapse on the principal neurons of the striatum, **medium-sized (not large), densely spiny neurons** (MSNs) which, depending on the species, account for up to 97% of striatal neurons (Bolam, 2010).

So, we "start" in the cortex, but what does that mean more precisely?

> It had long been assumed that any particular region of the neocortex, for example, the motor cortex, sends the same cortical information to striatal projection neurons whether they belong to the direct pathway or to the indirect pathway (Graybiel, 2005).

I'm not sure what specific information comes from motor cortex (maybe a "command," but what *is* a command, and how is it coded?), never mind whether the same data transmit to different pathways.

Graybiel draws attention to findings in rats (Lei et al., 2004) regarding two types of corticostriatal projection neurons. The first group of neurons, called "**pyramidal tract type**," are found in lower layer V of motor cortex; they send main axons into the pyramidal tract, but, in addition, they send collaterals off the main axons to striatum. They synapse primarily on striatal neurons of the indirect pathway.

The second group of neurons, called "**intratelencephalically projecting type**," are found in layer III and upper layer V of motor cortex. Their axons project to ipsilateral striatum (often to contralateral striatum as well) and to other areas of cortex, but they never leave the telencephalon–they do not pass to brainstem. Within striatum, the intratelencephalically projecting axons arborize over a space of ~1.5 mm. The arbors involve mainly striatal neurons of the **direct pathway**. Graybiel thinks that the two different corticostriatal projections allow for indirect pathway striatal neurons to receive a corollary discharge of descending motor commands, whereas the direct pathway neurons receive something else, "a signal integrated with transcortical signaling."

Even as we head to striatum, we face the matter of direct or indirect routes and another issue: a motor command, whatever it may be neurophysiologically, could result from microcircuit processing either in cortex, subcortex, or, most likely, in both.

*

Work? Bolam (2010) characterizes what MSNs do: "The essential computation performed by the striatum is the selection of which MSNs will fire, the consequence of which is altered firing of basal ganglia output neurons and hence the selection of the basal ganglia-associated behavior." In "*Globus Pallidus,* **lateral** (in particular)," we learned that MSNs are generally quiet, even if they receive glutamatergic afferents from cortex.[13]

---

[13] Also in that chapter, we outlined the difference between a direct pathway (striatum to medial GP to thalamus) and an indirect pathway (striatum to lateral GP to STN to medial GP to thalamus). We can be utterly basic about both of them–and even about a third known pathway, called **hyperdirect** (cortex to STN to medial GP). All are paths within presumably closed loops

The nature of the work depends on other factors. I rely on Bolam's discussion, already cited, in the next section.

*

What's the weather like? "Weather" is a metaphor for the "outside" that influences travel.

How MSNs respond to excitatory drive relates to two types of inhibition acting on them. First, MSNs (which are GABAergic and inhibitory) send collaterals in the direction of other MSNs within a pathway, whether direct or indirect. The inhibitory collaterals don't synapse at the cell bodies of MSNs, but rather at a distance from the soma, along the spiny portions of dendrites. The inhibition is generally weak, but varies with the amount of collateral activation.

A second mechanism involves cortical (and thalamic) excitation of GABAergic interneurons, which account for three to ten percent of striatal neurons. The interneurons strongly inhibit large numbers of MSNs.[14]

Aside from cortical and thalamic afferents, there are the other projections to striatum, including dopamine in particular, but also histamine (from hypothalamus) and serotonin. Acetylcholine also influences striatum both by cholinergic projections to it–e.g., from **pedunculopontine nucleus**–and as a consequence of very large cholinergic interneurons that also populate striatum. The cumulative effect of these several neurotransmitters can be short or long term; Graybiel talks about how dopamine, for example, "teaches" the striatum in an ongoing way (Graybiel, 2005). See also **"Olfactory Tubercle."**

*

---

of the kind we discussed in **"Labeled Line"** and elsewhere (viz., pathways embedded in a general cortico-striatal-pallidal-thalamo-cortical circuit).

How the three pathways (hyperdirect, direct, indirect) might operate in a real-time sequence has been addressed by Nambu. 2002, though, in fairness, Mink and Thach discussed much the same issue years earlier (Mink and Thach, 1993).

[14] Inhibition, mediated by multiple types of interneurons, is a hallmark of cortical microcircuits as well (see Markam et al., 2004). It's tempting to think that basal ganglionic inhibition is different in degree but not in kind to inhibitions that sculpt cortical output.

Home? As important as the decision to go to work is the question of when to leave it. What's the temporal relationship between cortical and striatal activity?

The concept that striatum and its connections modulate cortically driven action raises the question, at least, of when it does so. Axons of pyramidal type neurons dispatch collaterals to striatum on their way to brainstem and spinal cord, so is cortex the driving force with striatum a side-loop matter? If so, what's to be made of work that suggests a role for striatum in action selection? See **"Sequences,"** but here's a preview, if the reader is reading sequentially through this book:

> Most work on the function of the striatum in action selection has been in the context of decision making, in which animals are rewarded for choosing from among a set of simple behavioral alternatives. However, the concept of action selection can include more probabilistic and naturalistic forms of behavior, such as sequence generation (Markowitz et al., 2018).

Attention to what happens when–at a moment in some action–doesn't speak to what role cortex plays in relation to striatum in real time. Why would cortex be involved at all in what could be considered automatic action sequences? For example, if not asked specifically about it, are we conscious of how many times a minute we blink our eyes?

In a well-learned task involving sequential saccades, Fujii and Graybiel (2005) recorded simultaneously from cortex and striatum in two monkeys. Graybiel, writing separately about that study, distills the results:

> The activity of the striatum could either lead or lag that of cortex, or the two could have nearly simultaneous activation, depending on what part of the task the monkeys were performing, what the cognitive and motor demands of the task were, and what cortical area was monitored.... [T]here is not a fixed timing relationship between the neural activities in the neocortex and those in striatum in neural activities between cortex and striatum (Graybiel, 2005).

Based on the above findings, a better concept than modulation (which suggests basal ganglia as always *post hoc* to cortex) would be some process more streamingly live: "the production of circuit variability needed for on-line corrections of already learned behaviors" (Graybiel, 2005).

You go home and head to work. The back and forth is variable in time and in real life.[15]

---

[15] On the issue of timing, I find Mink (who wrote many papers with his mentor, Thach) instructive (1996):

> The types of neuronal activity in the putamen during limb movement can be divided into several groups. One pattern of activity is time-locked to movement and occurs during the movement. A second pattern follows an instructional cue and precedes movement. This type of activity is thought to be related to the intent or "set" of the animal and is often referred to as set-related activity. A third type of activity is related to movement occurring in the context of prior movements or specific task conditions. Finally, some striatal neurons fire in relation to specific sensory stimuli, usually when the stimulus is presented in the context of a movement.

See "**Sequences.**"

15.

Nucleus accumbens septi

I had wanted to meet him during his lifetime, to express admiration for prose that's instructive without evidence of any effort whatsoever. Judge for yourself; Nauta likely wrote the following himself, though he coauthored his textbook with Feirtag:

> ... the caudate nucleus and the putamen meet at the ventral limit of the capsule. (In fact, they meet through the triangular gap in the cone of the internal capsule.) The zone of confluence is called the nucleus accumbens, or, more elaborately, the nucleus accumbens septi: the nucleus leaning against the septum ... (Nauta and Feirtag, 1986).

We visualize a coronal section anterior to the anterior commissure:

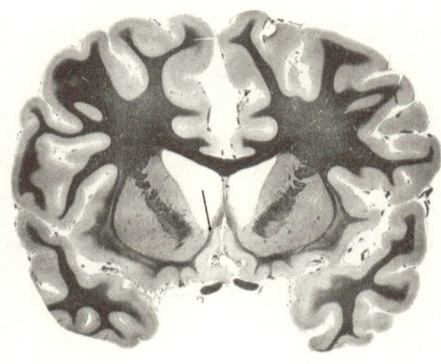

The arrow (just on one side) points to a white matter structure, along which the *nucleus accumbens septi* indeed seems to lean. The white matter is in the area of the midline ***septum pellucidum***, but why is it so visibly dark in this section stained for myelin?

The arrow indicates the ***rostrum* of *corpus callosum***, to be distinguished from other parts of the anterior third of *corpus callosum*, including the **genu** and the "**rostral body**" (the latter is part of "body of *corpus callosum*" that forms the roof of the frontal horns of lateral ventricle). The *rostrum*, however, sits deep and posterior to the callosum's genu. (The genu itself can be found in a coronal section anterior to one we use.)

*

Back to Nauta:

> . . . the nucleus accumbens, along with much, perhaps even all, of the caudate nucleus, receives input from the limbic system. Indeed, it receives substantial direct projections from both of the limbic "head ganglia," the hippocampus and the amygdala. Thus, there is reason to divide the striatum into a region under multiple limbic influence and a region receiving much sparser limbic input. The neocortical afferentation of the striatum obeys this parcellation in a curious way. The nucleus accumbens and the rest of the "limbic striatum" get their neocortical input from frontal association cortex–from the most nearly limbic part of the neocortex, one might say (Nauta and Feirtag, 1986).

In one sentence a bit later, he summarizes: "One begins to find it strange that the corpus striatum is taken merely to be motoric."

*

There's a developmental aspect to consider in light of Nauta's teaching. "Striatum" and all the names under that catch-term, including, *nucleus accumbens septi*, olfactory tubercle, caudate, putamen, **caudatoputamen**, neostriatum, **paleostriatum, ventral striatum, limbic striatum**, etc.,

generate basically correct thoughts that 1. *all* striatum arises from a periventricular "mantle" layer that eventually develops into eminences (see "**Eminences**"), and that, 2. complex neuronal migration to final positions follows.

But both thoughts need to be supplemented by a grander observation, corroborated in study of human fetuses before the tenth week of gestation, that the appearance of structures such as,

hypothalamus,
median forebrain bundle,
hippocampus,
amygdaloid complex,
mesencephalic tegmentum,
septal area,
stria terminalis,
and *nucleus accumbens septi*,

happens in an intimate developmental (temporal and spatial) relationship between sites (Müller and O'Rahilly, 2006).
See "**Bed Nuclei of *Stria Terminalis*,**" "**Infundibulum**," "**Juxtallocortical Connection (to Hypothalamus)**," "**Olfactory Tubercle**," and "**Quadrilateral Space of Broca**."

*

Finally, the anatomic proximity of *nucleus accumbens* and rostrum underscores an association to which we will return: rostrum links **orbitofrontal cortices** in either hemisphere, among other frontal locales in both hemispheres (Sakai et al., 2017), and orbitofrontal cortex projects to limbic striatum. The association, to be clear, is between special domains of striatum and what Nauta called "the most nearly limbic part of the neocortex."
See "**Projections of the Striasomal System**."

16.

Olfactory Tubercle

It may seem odd to spend any time writing about a structure that Nieuwenhuys et al. (2008d) thought was ambiguous and enigmatic even in animals with a decent sense of smell. Interest begins with the name, because, yes, the olfactory tubercle is involved in olfaction, yet it's a striatal structure.

*

Here's Switzer et al., writing about 40 years ago (in 1982):

> One of the distinguishing characteristics of the neocortex, as opposed to the rest of the cortical mantle, i.e., the allocortex, is generally thought to be its prominent projections to the corpus striatum. . . . [I]t has been proposed that the allocortex, like the neocortex, is closely related to the striato-pallidal system. According to this concept, the allocortex (hippocampus and piriform cortex [though some might say that piriform cortex, in an anatomically strict sense, is rhinencephalic, not allocortical]) projects to the ventral parts of the corpus striatum in the same way as the neocortex projects to the main dorsal parts of the corpus striatum.

It *is* a distinguishing characteristic of cortex that it projects prominently to *corpus striatum*, yet I wonder whether most people these days would argue that cortex's primary characteristic *just isn't* its connectivity with basal ganglia. I wonder why not. The obvious should be re-stated when people don't heed the obvious.

If allocortex, in a general sense (i.e., any cortex *other* [*allos*] than neocortex), links to the striato-pallidal system, then, the authors say, it's time "for a redefinition of some of the more prominent forebrain structures, including the ***substantia innominata*** and the olfactory tubercle." They were right 40 years ago, as they are today.

*

What area do we discuss?

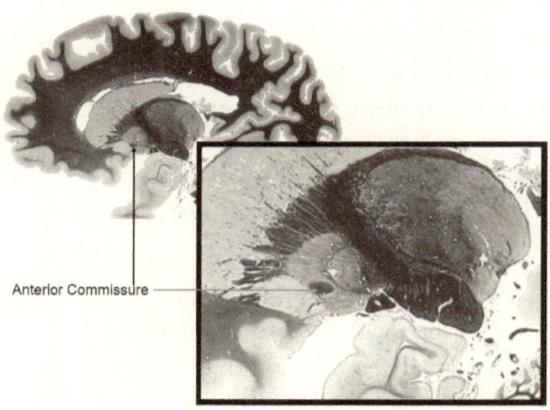

Anterior commissure is a landmark; I indicate its location with a black arrow in the parasagittal whole brain cut and with a grey arrow in the magnified inset. If we follow the grey arrow from left to right, we pass through a light area of striatum. Surrounding the commissure is a darker area, which is *globus pallidus*. Ventral to the level of the anterior commissure, then, we find *ventral* striatal and pallidal structures. The olfactory tubercle is part of ventral striatum, as is a portion of *nucleus accumbens septi*.

Switzer et al.'s seminal work demonstrated in detail how striatum and pallidum extend into the space of the basal forebrain (see "**Quadrilateral Space of Broca**"). The authors talk about just a part of olfactory tubercle being striatal. The whole olfactory tubercle, which isn't conspicuous in human brains, sits at the very base of the olfactory tract as the latter bifurcates into medial and lateral striae in the basal forebrain. The tubercle is more obvious in other mammals than humans, except microsmatic dolphins and whales.

A cortex-striatum relationship as well as influences on that system (see **"Macro-, Microcircuitry"**) are captured in a *précis* in the small anatomical space of basal forebrain.

Microscopically, the tubercle consists of three layers. The most ventral (superficial or closest to pia mater) of the three receives input from olfactory bulb. The middle layer dorsal to it is dense with medium spiny neurons–MSNs just as one would find in nucleus accumbens or in neostriatum, though MSNs are present in all three layers of the tubercle. In the most dorsal and thickest (deepest) layer, one observes tight clusters of neurons (called the **islands of Calleja**) that are particularly rich in choline acetyltransferase and acetylcholinesterase (Cansler et al., 2020).

We can summarize the tubercle's neurochemical mosaic, based on work mostly in rats; major sources of each transmitter, neuromodulator, or hormone are in parentheses (Cansler et al., 2020):

GABA (MSNs of olfactory tubercle)
Glutamate (projections from **olfactory bulb** and
piriform cortex [rhinencephalon])
Dopamine (ventral tegmental area of Tsai via
the median forebrain bundle)[16]
Acetylcholine (interneurons within olfactory tubercle, islands
of Calleja, projections via **diagonal band of Broca**)
Norepinephrine (*locus ceruleus* projections via median forebrain bundle)
Serotonin (raphe nuclei projections via median forebrain bundle)

---

[16] Dopamine projections may co-release glutamate (Hnasko et al., 2010). Dopaminergic innervation targets both MSNs and the islands of Calleja. Ventral tegmental area (of Tsai) is a dopaminergic nucleus as is the *pars compacta* of *substantia nigra*. Individual dopaminergic neurons have been observed to form widely spread and dense arbors at terminal locations (Matsuda et al., 2009). The arbors spread so widely that they seem to innervate different compartments or elements within striatum (e.g., MSNs as well as the islands of Calleja in the olfactory tubercle or, as Matsuda et al. specifically studied, matriosomal and striosomal compartments in neostriatum). See **"Projections of the Striasomal System."**

Estrogen (*in situ* in olfactory tubercle)
Endogenous opioids (*in situ* in olfactory tubercle)
Oxytocin (supraoptic and paraventricular nuclei of hypothalamus).

The list is incomplete, as Cansler et al. acknowledge. The point, however, is that in rhinencephalon and ventral striatum, there's a cortico-striatal-pallidal organization under various influences due to projections *not* from cortex, striatum, or pallidum. Amazingly as well, there's *in situ* neuromodulation (e.g., by estrogen produced in olfactory tubercle). A projection from ventral pallidum to mesio- (or medio-) dorsal thalamus has been reported (Zahm and Heimer, 1987), but smell is unlike the other senses in that olfactory *cortex* projects itself to thalamus (not the inverse), and medial thalamus projects, in turn, to frontal association cortex. Nevertheless, cortico-striatal-pallidal-thalamo-cortical circuitry again emerges as a leitmotif in our discussion.

17.

Projections of the Striasomal System

The original report describing a visually *in*homogeneous striatum in human, rhesus, and feline brains, based on staining for acetylcholinesterase, dates to 1978 (Graybiel and Ragsdale, 1978). The authors describe their findings carefully:

> ... pale zones never appeared completely free of enzyme activity and exhibited at least a weak cholinesterase reaction that made it easy to distinguish them from outlying fiber bundles of the internal capsule [which don't stain at all] . . . .. The borders of the pale zones were not crisp . . . .. Occasionally, however, the background stain at the borders of a pale zone appeared especially dense, as though a rim of more concentrated enzyme surrounded the region of low activity.

Staining for an enzyme involved in cholinergic neurotransmission doesn't prove the presence of, say, cholinergic interneurons in the striatum, but those do exist (see **"Macro-, Microcircuitry"**). The interneurons are very large, aspiny, and although they account for a minority of neurons within striatum, their effect on the vastly greater number of medium-sized, densely spiny neurons is widespread.

The word **"striasome"** doesn't appear in the 1978 report. The dark-staining background is called a **"matrix"** just once. The authors wonder whether their visualization of patchiness in two dimensions might not describe the 3D reality of what they see. Eventually, the words "striasome" (pale staining striatal bodies) and "**matrisome**" (patchy zones *within* dark-staining matrix–we'll address the latter momentarily) enter the neuroscience vocabulary and they stay in play for years:

> Striosomes and matrisomes are three-dimensionally labyrinthine structures spread out widely within the striatum, not local patches or spheres. Moreover, the striosomes have distributions suggesting that they could provide nearly complete coverage of the part of the striatum in which they lie. This means that they could serve to coordinate, in space and time, the activity of many striatal neurons within their resident regions (Graybiel, 2018).

If a given labyrinth is as extensive as the above description attests, it may not be that striasomes work in any kind of silo within striatum. Their effects would be distributed, not local.

*

As we've done previously, we can follow inputs into the striatal system (this next selection concentrates on **primary sensory cortex**, or "SI (the Roman numeral "I")," although much the same applies to primary motor cortex as it projects to striatum):

> Any one small part of the body map in SI projects to multiple, partly interconnected zones in the sensorimotor striatum. Such zones have been called matrisomes to indicate that they are patchy zones in the matrix compartment of the striatum, and to distinguish them from the patchy zones that form the chemically distinct striosomes. Different body part representations are sent to different sets of input matrisomes, though closely related body part projections may overlap. *Thus the information sent from SI to striatum is topographically specified but is broadly distributed* [authors' italics] (Graybiel and Kimura, 1985).

Next, from the same source:

> Striatal neurons projecting to each segment of the globus pallidus have a clumpy arrangement. Individual neurons project to one segment or to the other, but some neurons projecting to the external segment of the globus pallidus [lateral GP] are intermingled with those projecting to the internal segment [medial GP]; i.e., [lateral GP]-projecting matrisomes and [medial GP]-projecting matrisomes overlap. *This arrangement suggests that there may be a modular "template" in the striatum for redistributing information to the pallidum, and that there is provision for sending matched signals to [lateral GP and medial GP]* [authors' italics].

The important thing to notice is that striosomes don't factor into the discussion. The reason is simple and almost counterintuitive: projections to the matrisomal system are somatosensory and somatomotor, period.

You have to follow other cortical projections to get to striosomes. In 1985, the other projections are called generically limbic (in a broad sense that includes amygdala, hippocampus, and the diencephalic-and-brainstem "limbic continuum").

In a review from 2018, Graybiel narrows the discussion to rostral **cingulate gyrus** and caudal orbitofrontal cortex, and, she adds:

> ... neurons in striosomes project to the immediate vicinity of the dopamine-containing neurons of the [*substantia nigra pars compacta*], as well as directly to some of the dopamine-containing neurons,[17] and they project to lateral habenula [see "**Habenula**"], where they can further influence responses to both negative and positive stimuli (Graybiel, 2018).

---

[17] There's good reason why Graybiel makes the distinction between "the immediate vicinity" of a dopaminergic neuron and the neuron itself. When the projections terminate "in the vicinity"–viz., at a dendrite–a most remarkable entwining mesh appears. It looks like a floral bouquet. By confocal imaging, these bouquets are beautiful, in very vivid color (I don't reproduce it in this book's black-white-grey format). Please consult the reference, which is Crittenden et al., 2016.

The upshot is that if we're going to teach meaningfully about subcortical output in the future, we probably should broaden our scope to include *substantia nigra pars compacta* as an *output* nucleus *of striatum*, just as we say that medial GP is an output nucleus from the basal ganglia (see "***Ansa lenticularis***"). Traditionally, we think about a midbrain-*to*-striatal pathway (see "**Olfactory Tubercle**"), but the times . . . they're a-changing.

18.

Quadrilateral Space of Broca

Why Broca chose a donkey's brain for his illustration, I can't say. But here is his figure 48 from 1888; it depicts the ventral surface of a whole left hemibrain:

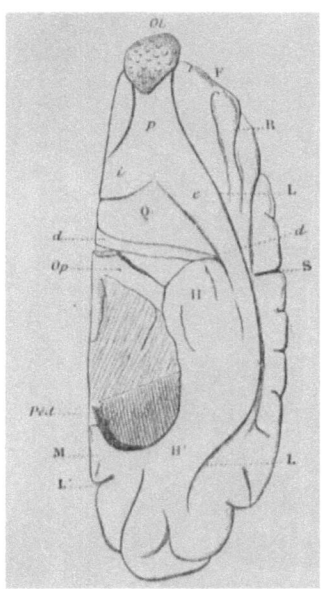

The space marked by "Q" has the following limits or boundaries: anterolaterally, what Broca called the external olfactory root (the **lateral olfactory stria**); the acute angle form by that stria and "where it meets the hippocampus" (marked "H"); a diagonal band that marks the posterior extent of the space (what we'd now call the **horizontal limb of the diagonal band of Broca**; its **vertical limb** tracks along the medial brain); the medial interhemispheric midline; then the **medial olfactory stria** anteromedially.

The chapter's question is elementary: what's deep to the quadrilateral space?

*

For a specific reason, the type of vertebrate animal's brain that I'll choose to help us with an answer will be marsupial–specifically, the brain of *Didelphis virginiana*, or the North American opossum, in an anterior coronal section:

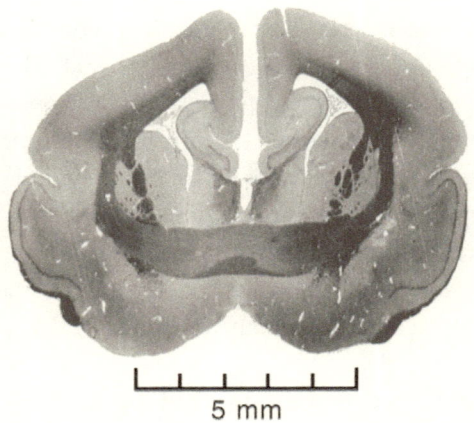

The specific reason is that all marsupial brains have *no corpus callosum*, so there's zero chance to confuse big, transverse white matter tracts in the anterior brain. In the marsupial, the thick anterior tract traversing the hemispheres can only be anterior commissure. Ventral to that commissure are structures most immediately deep to Broca's quadrilateral space.

*

The opossum section disorients the human neuroanatomist for reasons aside from an absence of *corpus callosum*, as I'll try to illustrate with textbook help (Hamel, 1982):

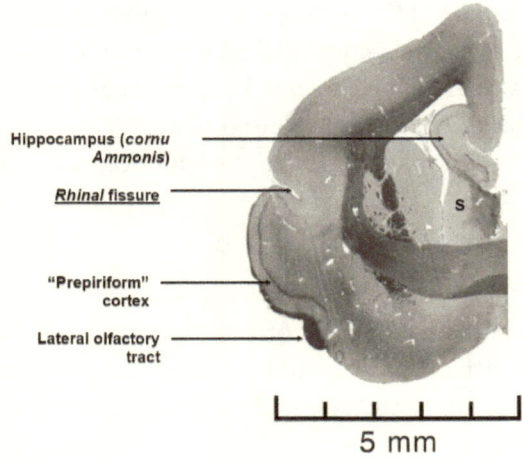

A first observation is that the hippocampal complex–**dentate gyrus** and *cornu Ammonis*–*isn't* in medial *temporal* lobe. (I address the medialness of hippocampus at greater length in *Teaching Hippocampal Anatomy*.) Second, the lateral fissure marked as "rhinal" is a length-wise fissure visible on the opossum brain's lateral surface that extends from very front to very back; it separates a dorsal pallium from a ventral, rhinencephalic, "prepiriform" cortex. Third, the lateral olfactory tract, analogous to the human (or donkey) lateral olfactory stria, is darkly prominent. And medial to it is . . . olfactory tubercle, which bulges ventrally. (See **"Olfactory Tubercle."**)

One also notes grey matter, marked by an "S," ventral to the hippocampal complex and medial to the head of caudate: it is a medial septal nucleus–a structure in the opossum brain that puts one in mind of medial projections from septal cholinergic nuclei in humans (Selden et al., 1998). But in humans, the well-known cholinergic *nucleus basalis* of Meynert occupies space *ventral* to anterior commissure; indeed it's a major structure within the *"substantia innominata* [of Karl Reichert, who, in studying cell groups of the basal forebrain, reportedly forgot to name tissue under *globus pallidus*]" or "**anterior perforated substance** [so named because of little holes created by penetrating vessels through the ventral surface]." Both are standard textbook terms that refer, simply, to Broca's quadrilateral space.

*

If we think next about structures hugging the **interhemispheric fissure**, we have the following, all dorsal to the anterior commissure: hippocampal complex, medial septal nucleus, and, then: medial to the medial septal nucleus buried within in white matter that seems to arise from hippocampus, there's a **nucleus of the diagonal band of Broca** (in the vertical limb of the band). Ventral to the anterior commissure we can say, not too simplistically, that we have obvious ventral striatum.

*

If at any time, you're at a loss thinking about structures that link to each other in the basal forebrain,[18] I invite consideration of alternative, vertebrate brains. In the marsupial especially, a "greater limbic system" really does look like an anatomically medial system of forebrain. See **"Juxtallocortical Connection (to Hypothalamus)."**

---

[18] Consider a sentence such as this: "The basal forebrain is composed of an affiliation of structures, including the medial septum, ventral pallidum, vertical diagonal band and horizontal diagonal band nuclei, substantia innominata/extended amygdala, and peripallidal regions; these structures contain a heterogeneous mixture of cell types that differ in transmitter content, morphology, and projection pattern (Zaborszky and Gombkoto, 2018)." With the exception of "peripallidal regions," which refer to collections of neurons around ventral pallidum that seem to co-locate with portions of nucleus basalis of Meynert (in study of feline brains; Jayaraman, 1983), all the structures mentioned organize themselves perhaps more clearly in the opossum image. The coronal section I chose is anterior to both the ventral pallidum and amygdala.

19.

Reticular Nucleus of Thalamus

An image, in which we can visualize it well, is a Nissl stain of a coronal section of an owl monkey's brain (*Aotus trivigatus*):[19]

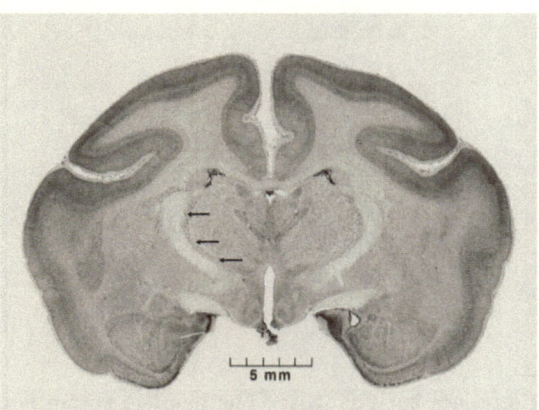

One has to be precise about what the arrows indicate (they're placed only on the left side of the image); I consulted a source regarding *Aotus* coronal section anatomy (Stepniewska et al., 1994) to corroborate what I write.

Since the stain reveals dark cells (white matter tracts are white), the arrows point to a curvilinear grey band at the lateral extreme of thalamus, just medial to the (white) **internal capsule**. The arrows specifically don't

---

[19] A human coronal section, similarly stained, doesn't reveal the structure as clearly.

point to internal capsule itself, which is immediately lateral to reticular nucleus in most all *Aotus* coronal sections through thalamus. Previously (see "**Diencephalon**, embryology of"), we mentioned a thalamic external medullary lamina, which derives from the *zona limitans intrathalamicus* (ZLI); the external medullary lamina is just medial to reticular nucleus, but I can't see well it in this section with its particular stain.

An ongoing theme in this monograph is the subcortex and inhibition, and reticular nucleus is yet another inhibitory center. We know that many GABAergic afferents arise from outside thalamus (see "*Ansa lenticularis*"), so what's the role of thalamic reticular nucleus if afferents to a "**basal-ganglia-recipient thalamus**" are already inhibitory (Goldberg et al., 2013)?

*

Let's peek at a network analysis conducted with respect to rat thalamus. The investigators divided thalamus into epithalamus (see "**Habenula**" regarding its two nuclei) and ventral and dorsal thalami, the last being the largest in terms of both volume "and the number of its grey matter regions (39 out of the 46 for the complete thalamus on each side of the brain)" (Swanson et al., 2019). Note, though, that their "ventral thalamus" refers *only* to five structures (reticular nucleus, a portion of lateral geniculate nucleus, the "intergeniculate leaflet," *zona incerta*, and the fields of Forel); they're specifically not referring to ventrally located nuclei such as ventroanterior or ventrolateral nucleus *inter alia*. Take Swanson et al. at their word, that reticular nucleus is "ventral thalamic," though there's debate about its precise embryologic origin (Halassa and Acsády, 2016; Puelles and Rubenstein, 2003).

As of 2019, according to Swanson et al., reticular nucleus was known to project to 32 of the 39 dorsal thalamic nuclei; 35 of the 39 dorsal thalamic nuclei have been shown to project to it. (Reticular nucleus is GABAergic, but most dorsal thalamic nuclei are glutamatergic. Axon collaterals of glutamatergic projections within thalamus innervate reticular nucleus.) By the authors' numbers, reticular nucleus alone accounts for about 60% of all ipsilateral intrathalamic connectivity. Another specialist has said outright that reticular nucleus is "the only hub with heavy intrathalamic connections" (Takata, 2019). In other words, as has been observed for some time (well before this decade), reticular nucleus receives input from most ipsilateral thalamic nuclei and, in turn, it projects back to most ipsilateral thalamic nuclei.[20]

Reticular nucleus projects *only* to thalamic nuclei. Does that fact call to mind a feature of medial pallidal output to thalamus?

The issue is unidirectionality. Halassa and Acsády are explicit on the subject: if, for example, medial pallidal output is unidirectional to thalamus, then its own activity isn't influenced by thalamic activity; there's no return call from thalamus to medial *globus pallidus*.[21] On the other hand, if reticular neurons only project to thalamic nuclei–to virtually all of them, no less–, then their activity, based on interaction with all thalamic nuclei, potentially has widespread thalamic effects, some of which we can observe for ourselves (honestly).

Reticular nucleus "allows the emergence of local reverberating oscillations [e.g., those that give rise to sleep spindles in an EEG of light sleep]," whereas pallidothalamic connections "may initiate but cannot maintain reverberating thalamic activity, . . . [but] may communicate long-term changes in cortical outputs as an inhibitory signal back to widespread cortical regions via the highly divergent axonal arbor of their thalamic

---

[20] As an aside, reticular neurons have quite unique features. In the following excerpt (Halassa and Acsády, 2016), "TRN" abbreviates "thalamic reticular nucleus":

> Adjacent TRN neurons can be electrically coupled by gap junctions, enabling coordinated firing. Moreover, gap junctions display activity-dependent plasticity that can dynamically alter their scale of action. Although the available evidence suggests that gap junctions exist only among closely spaced TRN cells, the extent to which electrical coupling varies within and between subnetworks is unclear. In the somatosensory TRN, most of gap junction (i.e., dye-) coupled TRN cells project to a single nucleus, probably enhancing focal subnetwork action, but in certain cases, dye-coupled cells can target two nuclei.

> We're about to make the point that reticular neurons project *only* to other thalamic nuclei, but it's also unique to reticular nucleus, as opposed to other thalamic nuclei, that it receives layer 6 cortical projections (glutamatergic) from virtually all cortical areas, aside from its intrathalamic connections.

[21] We'll discuss the point about "no return calls" elsewhere–see "***Zona incerta.***"

targets" (Halassa and Acsády, 2016). With a little training, you, too, can see a sleep spindle in an EEG during light sleep, plain as day.

Choose the inhibitory pathway you like (the pallidothalamic projection or the projections of reticular nucleus of thalamus within thalamus); the downstream effects will differ in the long-term course of life or during a night's early sleep.

20.

Sequences

I'll address the series of tones that constitute birdsong. After zebra finches hatch, they *acquire* song. So, actually, we discuss two sequences: 1. the tonal series of a song and 2. the sequential stages of the bird's learning, including "subsong" or babble, then an intermediate "plastic song," then birdsong itself. There's a critical period during which the birds copy a tutor song; there's variability at first, then stereotyped performance, "as all of us who enjoy bird songs know" (Graybiel, 2005).

Let's concentrate on work by Goldberg and Fee (2012), then think about the implications.

*

I'll simplify the authors' method and findings. A circuit involving anterior forebrain and specific thalamic and pallidal locales is known to be essential in a songbird vocalization (Olveczky et al., 2005). Goldberg and Fee (2012) interrogated the pathway by quantifying thalamic nuclear discharge in relation to pallidal neuronal firing in the babble or subsong of young zebra finches. Pallidal and thalamic neurons, recorded simultaneously, both fired during babbling and before subsong syllable onset.

The paradox, in their view, was that pallidal inhibition (pallidal firing) should briefly pause, so as to disinhibit thalamus. They next lesioned pallidum bilaterally only to find that song-locked thalamic firing persisted. Then they antidromically identified anterior forebrain neurons associated with the thalamic nucleus under study, and found that corticothalamic neurons activated during singing and before subsong syllable onset.

Their conclusion was that behavior-locked activity may be driven by cortical input to the basal-ganglia-recipient motor thalamus. See "**Thalamocortex.**"

What about mature song? Elsewhere (Goldberg et al., 2013) the investigators opine:

> In a variety of model systems, including songbirds and humans, BG [basal ganglia] lesions block the behavioral improvements that normally come with practice, and it is widely believed that the BG implements reinforcement learning to mediate the acquisition of motor skills. More specifically, there is evidence that the BG provides the thalamus with a premotor signal that biases motor output towards improved performance. The end result of learning is, in essence, taking the right action in the right context (or at the right time in a motor sequence) . . ..

One can access audio of zebra finch song; it makes for pleasant background noise while working. Without listener training, however, one can't be certain about the type of birdsong one hears—whether babble, plastic, or mature song. More than that, it's as if one listens *blindly*, without being able even to distinguish zebra finch from other birdsong.

The situation with more familiar music differs, of course. I like Mozart and Bach; if given a piece of music by one or the other, I think I could tell the difference between the two within moments.[22] Do the sequences of notes (right actions in right contexts) give away the difference? Partly perhaps, but I'm not sure completely. It seems to me that parsing any music has to do with more than the notes. Bach and Mozart *are just* different.

*

---

[22] I mean J.S. Bach, not (for example) J.C. Bach, who was J.S.B.'s eleventh son among an astonishing eighteen total children. J.C.B.'s lightheartedness (the so-called *galant* style) certainly influenced Mozart, but I'd argue that even J.C.B. is distinguishable from *Amadé*, the French moniker that Leopold Mozart's son much preferred, as opposed to either Wolfgang or Amadeus or Christostomos (the last being one of Mozart's several names given to him at his baptism).

I lurch towards my meaning. The birdsong work points to an issue about the timescales of sequences. We can accept as a given that there's different noise generated by newly hatched birds vs. adults–it's a matter of a developmental timescale for zebra finches.

After onset of song then the ensuing music, at what point (one bar? two notes?) does one know that Bach or Mozart is playing, or whether the musician who plays them is skilled or tedious?

It's at the micro level of analyzing sequences that we're learning how cortex and subcortex work in concert.[23]

The italicized sentence finds support in work looking at the "syllables" that comprise a rat's physical movements in space. What the syllables are (rearing on hind legs as opposed to forward movement with all four, etc.) isn't quite the interest here; the notable finding is that cortical-subcortical pathways thought to operate in counterpoint to each other may not *apparently* work that way based on evidence, until one applies an appropriate timeframe for analysis:

> When averaged over timescales of single syllables, we observe strong correlations in direct and indirect pathway activity across most behavioral syllables. However, when viewed at the sub-syllable timescale, many syllables exhibit periods in which decorrelations between [direct-pathway spiny projection neurons of striatum] and [indirect spiny projection neurons of striatum] are apparent. From both an encoding and decoding perspective these decorrelations appear to play an important role in conveying information about the identity and form of individual behavioral syllables (Markowitz et al., 2018).

(It's as if you ascertain a difference in composers inside the interval between a couple of notes.) Moment-to-moment analysis differs from syllable analysis. A syllable lasts a while; pathway activities are distinguishable only at sub-syllable time intervals.

---

[23] The point is not lost upon Goldberg et al. (2013). When analyzed in very short time intervals, relations between firing trains revealed that pallidal inputs were very inhibitory, but "the duration of this inhibitory pulse during singing was extremely brief (~5 ms)," and the effect on thalamus also depended on the pallidal *interspike* interval, which, though variable, also measured in microseconds.

21.

Thalamocortex

Cortical "afferentation" (Luria's term; see "**Diencephalon**, embryology of") happens by multiple channels. If we wanted to count how many channels in total (we wouldn't finish, alas), we could start with thalamus.

*

In "**Reticular Nucleus of Thalamus**," we heard about 46 grey matter regions in a single rat thalamus. Rats aren't humans, but we could work through all the regions, so as to organize them, roughly, in relationship to cortex. Here they all are, organized alphabetically by the abbreviations used in Swanson, 2019:

AD	ANTERODORSAL THALAMIC NUCLEUS
AM d	ANTEROMEDIAL THALAMIC NUCLEUS DORSAL PART
AM v	ANTEROMEDIAL THALAMIC NUCLEUS VENTRAL PART
AV	ANTEROVENTRAL THALAMIC NUCLEUS
CL	CENTRAL LATERAL THALAMIC NUCLEUS
CM	CENTRAL MEDIAL THALAMIC NUCLEUS
FF	FIELDS OF FOREL
IAD	INTERANTERODORSAL THALAMIC NUCLEUS

IAM	INTERANTEROMEDIAL THALAMIC NUCLEUS
IGL	INTERGENICULATE LEAFLET
IMD	INTERMEDIODORSAL THALAMIC NUCLEUS
LD	LATERAL DORSAL THALAMIC NUCLEUS
LG d	DORSAL LATERAL GENICULATE NUCLEUS
LG v	VENTRAL LATERAL GENICULATE NUCLEUS
LH	LATERAL HABENULA
LP	LATERAL POSTERIOR THALAMIC NUCLEUS, rat homologue of human **pulvinar**
MD c	MEDIODORSAL THALAMIC NUCLEUS CENTRAL PART
MD l	MEDIODORSAL THALAMIC NUCLEUS LATERAL PART
MD m	MEDIODORSAL THALAMIC NUCLEUS MEDIAL PART
MG d	MEDIAL GENICULATE COMPLEX DORSAL PART
MG m	MEDIAL GENICULATE COMPLEX MEDIAL PART
MG v	MEDIAL GENICULATE COMPLEX VENTRAL PART
MH	MEDIAL HABENULA
PCN	PARACENTRAL THALAMIC NUCLEUS
PF	PARAFASCICULAR NUCLEUS
PO	POSTERIOR THALAMIC COMPLEX
POL	POSTERIOR LIMITING THALAMIC NUCLEUS
PP	PERIPEDUNCULAR NUCLEUS
PR	PERIREUNIENS NUCLEUS
PT	PARATENIAL NUCLEUS
PVT	PARAVENTRICULAR THALAMIC NUCLEUS
RE c	NUCLEUS REUNIENS CAUDAL DIVISION
RE r	NUCLEUS REUNIENS ROSTRAL DIVISION
RH	RHOMBOID NUCLEUS
RT	RETICULAR NUCLEUS
SGN	SUPRAGENICULATE NUCLEUS

SMT	SUBMEDIAL THALAMIC NUCLEUS
SPF m	SUBPARAFASCICULAR NUCLEUS MAGNOCELLULAR PART
SPF p	SUBPARAFASCICULAR NUCLEUS PARVICELLULAR PART
VAL	VENTRAL ANTERIOR-LATERAL THALAMIC COMPLEX
VM	VENTRAL MEDIAL THALAMIC NUCLEUS
VPL pc	VENTRAL POSTEROLATERAL THALAMIC NUCLEUS PARVICELLULAR PART
VPL pr	VENTRAL POSTEROLATERAL THALAMIC NUCLEUS PRINCIPAL PART
VPM pc	VENTRAL POSTEROMEDIAL THALAMIC NUCLEUS PARVICELLULAR PART
VPM pr	VENTRAL POSTEROMEDIAL THALAMIC NUCLEUS PRINCIPAL PART
ZI	ZONA INCERTA

To edit, let's: 1. Collapse parts or divisions of nuclei (so, for example: "VPL pc" and "VPL pr" become VPL; also, collapse "AD," "AM (d and v)," and "AV" into "anterior nuclei"); 2. Delete the two epithalamic/habenular nuclei and the "ventral" thalamic nuclei (for a list of five deemed "ventral," see **"Reticular Nucleus of Thalamus"**); 3. Collapse some nuclei which are "peri-," "supra-," or "sub-" to nuclei that we'll keep on the list (e.g., perireuniens nucleus goes out; *nucleus reuniens* remains; also, we'll think about suprageniculate nucleus as part of the posterior thalamic complex, PO); 4. Take out intralaminar nuclei and place them in a separate list (these are nuclei within the boundary of the internal medullary lamina of thalamus); 5. Take out midline nuclei and also place them in a separate list. Then we're left with a category of two "other" nuclei that are posterior and lateral in rat thalamus–their significance isn't clear to me. In making the edits, I consulted various sources (Jones, 1985; Thompson and Robertson, 1987; Groenewegen and Berendse, 1994; Krout et al., 2002; Park et al., 2017; Zhou et al., 2017; Swanson, 2018).

We end up with this:

"A" ANTERIOR NUCLEI
LD LATERAL DORSAL THALAMIC NUCLEUS
LG LATERAL GENICULATE NUCLEUS
LP LATERAL POSTERIOR THALAMIC NUCLEUS, rat homologue of human pulvinar
MD MEDIODORSAL THALAMIC NUCLEUS
MG MEDIAL GENICULATE COMPLEX
PO POSTERIOR THALAMIC COMPLEX
VAL VENTRAL ANTERIOR-LATERAL THALAMIC COMPLEX
VM VENTRAL MEDIAL THALAMIC NUCLEUS
VPL VENTRAL POSTEROLATERAL THALAMIC NUCLEUS
VPM VENTRAL POSTEROMEDIAL THALAMIC NUCLEUS

INTRALAMINAR NUCLEI

CL CENTRAL LATERAL THALAMIC NUCLEUS
CM CENTRAL MEDIAL THALAMIC NUCLEUS
PCN PARACENTRAL THALAMIC NUCLEUS
PF PARAFASCICULAR NUCLEUS

MIDLINE NUCLEI[24]

IAD INTERANTERODORSAL THALAMIC NUCLEUS
IAM INTERANTEROMEDIAL THALAMIC NUCLEUS
IMD INTERMEDIODORSAL THALAMIC NUCLEUS

---

[24] Absolutely midline grey matter not included among Swanson's 46 nuclei would be *massa intermedia* or the **interthalamic adhesion**. Absent in 1/3 of men and 1/4 of women according to an older report, it can also disappear with age and brain atrophy (Lansdell and Davie, 1972). Its role in human cognition has been studied, but conclusions are uncertain: for example, why would presence of the adhesion be associated with subjective loneliness (Borghei et al., 2020)?

PT   PARATENIAL NUCLEUS
PVT PARAVENTRICULAR THALAMIC NUCLEUS
RE   NUCLEUS REUNIENS
RH   RHOMBOID NUCLEUS
SMT SUBMEDIAL THALAMIC NUCLEUS

OTHER (POSTEROLATERAL)[25]

POL POSTERIOR LIMITING THALAMIC NUCLEUS
PP   PERIPEDUNCULAR NUCLEUS

Does the first group look familiar? They include nuclei that we teach in introductory neuroanatomy.

Routine talk about sensory (VPL, VPM, the medial and lateral geniculate nuclei) and motor (VA/VL) nuclei misses an opportunity to characterize *all* thalamic nuclei, including those less often taught—particularly those in the intralaminar and midline groups.

*

Based on Sherman's work with coauthors (Sherman and Koch, 1998; Sherman and Guillery, 2002; Sherman, 2017), we can generate a list of principles to guide how to teach in a more advanced way than whatever we impart in the first or second year of medical school or in early neuroscience training.

1. All thalamic nuclei receive cortical input.
2. Except for reticular nucleus, all thalamic nuclei project to cortex (to its superficial layers).
3. Thalamic nuclei can receive bihemispheric input (e.g., Alloway et al., 2009 on the subject of bilateral whisker movements of the

---

[25] Both posterior limiting thalamic and peripeduncular nuclei are located near medial geniculate complex. Early investigators (Nissl, Gurdjian, Le Gros Clark) gave different names to these and other posterior nuclei, based on study specifically of rodents and other small mammals (Jones, 1985).

rat face), but "no contralateral efferent connections involving any thalamic nucleus have been found" (Sherman and Koch, 1998).[26]
4. Corticothalamic projections arise from layer 6 of cortex for all thalamic nuclei. Some, *not all*, thalamic nuclei also receive pyramidal projections from layer 5.
5. What distinguishes different thalamic nuclei is their respective subcortical *and* cortical afferentations.

To clarify the fourth point, think about the vertical leg of a right triangle and the triangle's hypotenuse:

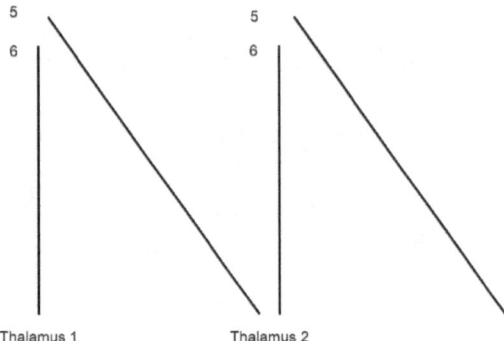

A hypotenuse represents a layer 5 projection to another thalamic nucleus (a "higher order" one). The arrangement allows for transthalamic transfer of information. We can speak of a "first order" connection between a thalamic nucleus and cortex ("Thalamus 1" receives from layer 6 and will project to layers superficial to layer 6). Then we notice a different kind of nucleus that receives both layer 5 and 6 cortical input ("Thalamus 2").

*

An example: trigeminal input projects to VPM; VPM projects to and receives input from primary sensory cortex; VPM is a first order nucleus.

Compare VPM to posterior nuclear complex (PO), which receives input from (and likely projects to) medial and lateral posterior parietal cortex *and* primary sensory cortex (Olsen and Witter, 2016). PO is "higher

---

[26] See, however, "**Uncrossed?**" for a discussion of Preuss and Goldman-Rakic, 1987.

order"–which may account for its role in complex aspects of sensation–e.g., the vexed issue of pain perception) (Masri et al., 2009).

Another example: cerebellar output directs to ventral anterior (VA) nucleus in what seems a first order connection. VA receives cortical input not only from primary motor cortex, but also, as discussed in "**Labeled Line**," from other, non-primary motor cortex, presumably from layer 5 pyramidal neurons. VA is "a mosaic," with both first order and higher order connectivity (Sherman, 2017).

Last example: Central medial nucleus (which is particularly developed in humans; it's the only intralaminar nucleus that's disproportionately large in primates compared to other non-primate species [Kemp and Powell, 1970]) receives afferents from basal ganglia, cerebellum, and spinal cord (Sherman and Koch, 1998). Nieuwenhuys et al. (2008b) say that central medial nucleus projects "diffusely," but they fall back to a terser claim that central median nucleus might preferentially target primary motor cortex. Sherman and Koch (1998) emphasize a difference between a *dense* projection to a tight locale (as in the case of VPM to primary sensory cortex) as opposed to *diffuse* projection to a large, ill-defined cortical domain, as is the case with central medial nucleus.

We'll remark only that central medial nucleus–indeed all the intralaminar and midline nuclei–don't seem either first order or mixed.

*

The likes of Jones, Sherman, and Nieuwenhuys haven't specified the following groups. I have, and while I could be wrong about a detail or two, the exercise demonstrates that a majority of nuclei *aren't* first order.

First Order (they receive massive subcortical input from a particular source; they do not receive layer 5 pyramidal output):

LG   LATERAL GENICULATE NUCLEUS
VPL VENTRAL POSTEROLATERAL THALAMIC NUCLEUS
VPM VENTRAL POSTEROMEDIAL THALAMIC NUCLEUS

Mixed (they may receive subcortical input from a major source, including basal ganglia; they project to other-than-primary cortices):

LP	LATERAL POSTERIOR THALAMIC NUCLEUS, rat homologue of human pulvinar[27]
MG	MEDIAL GENICULATE COMPLEX (its non-ventral parts project to non-primary auditory cortex)
PO	POSTERIOR THALAMIC COMPLEX
VAL	VENTRAL ANTERIOR-LATERAL THALAMIC COMPLEX
VM	VENTRAL MEDIAL THALAMIC NUCLEUS

Higher Order (they may receive subcortical inputs [emphasis on multiple inputs], but, basically, they serve as "conduit[s] for information transfer between cortical areas" [Sherman, 2017]):

"A"	ANTERIOR NUCLEI
LD	LATERAL DORSAL THALAMIC NUCLEUS
MD	MEDIODORSAL THALAMIC NUCLEUS

<u>INTRALAMINAR NUCLEI</u>
<u>MIDLINE NUCLEI</u>

*

---

[27] I hedge by putting pulvinar in the mixed (as opposed to higher order) category, but it's hard to overlook its rich projection to primary visual cortex, just as VP nuclei densely project to primary sensory cortex. Sherman and Guillery (2002) call pulvinar "largely a higher-order relay." And:

> In order to understand the nature of the messages that are relayed through the pulvinar region from one cortical area to another, we need to understand how these messages relate to the functional properties of the cortical layer-5 cells that innervate the relay cells of the pulvinar region from several different cortical areas, and how those properties, in turn, relate to the functional properties of the cortical areas that receive an innervation from the pulvinar region. To a significant extent, lack of agreement as to how the region should be subdivided has prevented a systematic study of connectivity patterns.

A reasonable question regarding transthalamic transfer of information by way of higher order nuclei would be: "can't cortex just talk to itself?"[28] A rejoinder goes as follows: many, "perhaps all," corticocortical connections are modulatory, and . . .

> . . . the transthalamic pathway can provide the main information transfer. Thus, the full impact of the thalamus may be much more than simply controlling flow of information from the periphery and from other parts of the brain to the cortex: it may remain an active partner in all cortical computations (Sherman and Guillery, 2002).

Also, "thalamocortex," as a synergism, reflects the anatomy. Simple as that.

See "**Wakefulness**."

---

[28] Cortex does, in fact, connect to itself. For a discussion, see three chapters on "connectivity" in *The Frontal Brain and Language*.

22.

Uncrossed?

Classical, idiopathic Parkinson's disease should present asymmetrically in its early natural history; a clinician wants to hear about onset perhaps only on one side, because that information helps her to diagnose correctly. And she'd infer, in a case of right hemibody onset of slowness, stiffness and tremor, that: 1. There's asymmetric loss of dopamine neurons, more in the left than the right *substantia nigra pars compacta*; and 2. If she were to obtain a dopamine transporter (DAT) study, she'd expect reduced DAT in the left compared to the right neostriatum, most noticeably so in left (less) vs. right putamen. She might then conclude that subcortex on one side deals only with homolateral cortex, and that there's no crossing of fibers from one neostriatum to contralateral cortex, in the spirit of what two thalamus experts have said (see **"Thalamocortex"**), that no one has yet found an efferent from one thalamus to the contralateral hemisphere.

As in the first monograph of the present series (*The Crossed Organization of Brains*), can we think a bit harder about decussation and non-decussation?

*

The plan in this chapter is to revisit the diagnostic scenario just described with a focus on relevant anatomy.

<u>*Relationship of nigral (pars compacta) cell loss and side of signs or symptoms in the body*</u>. The discovery of MPTP as a toxin that specifically damages nigral cells happened during my years in medical school, so studies that explored hemiparkinsonism following unilateral carotid injection of MPTP

into a hemisphere (in monkeys) hold more than historical interest for me; they influenced my career path. For the record, unilateral carotid infusion of MPTP results in hemiparkinsonism in the contralateral hemibody (Bankiewicz et al., 1986). The relationship between a surgical lesion of nigra on one side and manifestations in the contralateral body had been described years earlier (Carpenter and Peter, 1972).

All simplifications die a form of death in a literature review. Can we marshal evidence for a projection from one *substantia nigra pars compacta* to the contralateral brain? Sure: for example, Gerfen et al., 1982 and Consolazione et al., 1985. The first of the sources mentions significant bilateral nigral projections to ventromedial nuclei of thalamus (ventromedial nucleus is what we'd describe as a mixed order nucleus; see **"Thalamocortex"**); the second paper speaks to why crossed projections matter (e.g., from nigra to contralateral striatum): the "physiological meaning" of those projections has to do with transfer of sensorimotor information between hemispheres.

Back to the neurologist: she's not wrong in what she thinks; in terms of clinicopathologic correlation, she's likely right. But could basal ganglia disease in general be a problem with bicortical afferentation via subcortex?

*

Asymmetrical striatal DAT. Relevant to the expectation that left striatal dopamine DAT would be less compared to the right striatum in our neurologist's case, consider a study of 30 Parkinsonian patients with asymmetrical but bilateral disease (all at Hoehn and Yahr stage II); a comparison group included 15 age-matched controls (Martin-Bastida et al., 2019). They used the selective PET ligand ^{11}CPE2I to determine striatal DAT and a novel MR method to quantify neuromelanin in subdivisions of *substantia nigra*. Loss of nigral neuromelanin did associate with decreased striatal DAT, only on the side (of brain) most affected. Keep in mind, however, that all the patients had bilateral signs, despite clinical asymmetry in each case. Depigmentation *was also bilateral*, and the association between loss of nigral neuromelanin and decreased striatal DAT *didn't* manifest in the less affected brain. Why not?

"Striatal DAT tended to correlate with bradykinetic/rigid/axial severity while nigral neuromelanin correlated with disease duration, particularly within the nigra," the authors wrote. Mean disease duration among the patients was about 7 years.

So our neurologist is right again, but she's wrong if she thinks that nigral cell loss *equals* decreased striatal DAT, according to findings of the 2019 study. You can't necessarily predict a downstream effect based on known connectivity.

*

<u>Subcortex on one side deals only with cortex on that same side of brain</u>. Is she wholly correct in that surmise?

*

I am a card-carrying, veteran member of the *please*-whatever-you-do-keep-it-simple-and-above-all-*clear* school of pedagogy, but the plain truth is that, regarding connections between nodes–

>cortex,
>striatum,
>*globus pallidus*,
>thalamus,

–one can learn about projections from:

>cortex to *homotopic contralateral cortex* (Muakkassa and Strick, 1979; see **"Labeled Line"**);

>cortex to *contralateral striatum* (and claustrum) (Künzle, 1975, an early anterograde study; but Hedreen and DeLong MR (1991) had doubts about the finding; later the subject of crossed projections earned a review (Fame et al., 2011); then Innocenti et al. (2017) added to growing evidence for cortex-to-contralateral striatum connections, with pretty tractography pictures);

globus pallidus to contralateral thalamus (Hazrati and Parent, 1991);[29]

and, yes, contrary to our thalamus experts quoted in **"Thalamocortex,"** from thalamus to *contralateral cortex* (Preuss and Goldman-Rakic, 1987).

Regarding a striatal to contralateral pallidal connection, Tremblay and Filion (1989) stimulated striatum on one side in awake monkeys to induce both ipsi- and contralateral pallidal response. They thought that the contralateral pallidal response resulted from activation of a polysynaptic pathway; they didn't invoke a monosynaptic projection from striatum to contralateral *globus pallidus*.

*

Our neurologist's conclusion that subcortex on one side deals only (or mainly) with cortex on that same side isn't refuted by the above citations. But a "one hemisphere-one homolateral subcortex" view doesn't speak to what she wants to understand, after she makes her accurate diagnosis. She's also interested to learn something pertinent to both normal and disturbed movement.

Luria, advocate of afferentation in a whole brain, offers this:

> Human movements are performed only comparatively rarely by only *one* hand. As a rule they require the coordinated participation of *both* hands, and this coordination has different degrees of complexity. In some cases, the simplest, it takes the form of equal, allied movements in which both hands simultaneously perform the same actions. . . . In other cases, the great majority, the movements of the two hands are coordinated in a

---

[29] Cajal hypothesized a monosynaptic striatocortical projection in the late 19th century, though his idea had its critics. Jayaraman (1980) confirmed that they exist using retrograde tracing. The striatal cells of origin were large, probably not medium spiny neurons. He also observed retrograde labeling of globus pallidus neurons after large injections in cortex. Striatal and pallidal efferents in his study didn't cross to contralateral cortex.

more complex fashion, in which the master (right) hand performs the principal action and the subordinate (left) hand merely provides the optimal conditions under which the right hand can work, playing the role of a provider of the motor background.... Finally, the most complex types of movement of the two hands are those which are mutually opposite or reciprocally coordinated in character... (author's italics, 1973).

"Provider of the motor background" is an interesting concept, because what *isn't* part of the background? It's hard not to notice that a substantial part of the brain's afferentation is... *itself,* arising from both hemispheres and subcortices, if we abide by Luria's trenchant view about what movement is, in general.

23.

Vascular Organ of the *Lamina Terminalis*

When sensory physiologists talk about the first telencephalic processing of sensory input, they might think of synapses in olfactory bulb and retina (Shepherd et al., 2018), but perhaps they could add the vascular organ of the *lamina terminalis* to their list. The structure is otherwise known as the *organum vasculosum laminae terminalis* (OVLT).

I want to think about it as an unpaired sensory organ uniquely situated both inside and outside the brain:

> . . . the OVLT is bounded by fluid on two sides. The subarachnoid space called the **prechiasmatic cistern** lies immediately rostral to the OVLT so that this circumventricular organ is an isthmus bordered on two sides by cerebrospinal fluid. One part of the OVLT is "inside" the brain and the other is on the "outside" . . . (authors' italics, Johnson and Loewy, 1990).

This chapter isn't about all the circumventricular organs; indeed there's disagreement over their total number in different mammals (Duvernoy and Risold, 2007). True, there are shared features of the "organs" that are anatomically peri- or circumventricular–viz., their location *inside* a ventricular space (whether third or fourth), their lack of blood-brain barrier (inside the organs themselves), their rich vascularity, etc.

But, unlike the inward-facing **subcommisural organ** or *area postrema* (which protrude into third and fourth ventricular space, respectively), OVLT is Janus-faced by virtue of its location at the rostral extent of the third ventricle–i.e., *within* the lamina terminalis (see "**Diencephalon, embryology of**").

As in the microcircuitry of olfactory bulb or retina, OVLT receives "sensory" information and transforms it into neural code. OVLT is a study of afferentation in miniature, with twists.

*

Duvernoy and Risold (2007) describe OVLT's bidirectional face in the context of its vascularization, which arises on the pial surface from **preoptic arteries** in the prechiasmatic cistern:

> [The vascular organ] consists of a superficial capillary network which lines the deep fold of the lamina terminalis [on the "outside" of the brain] . . .. The deep network is formed of capillary loops issuing from the superficial network. In the cat, the top of these loops does not reach the ventricular surface which is bordered with a fine subependymal network.

Whether the ventricular ependymal layer/subependymal network allows for exchange between blood and cerebrospinal fluid is unclear, but Duvernoy and Risold believe that there is transfer of . . . some data.

So, what afferent information does OVLT process? (Please don't reach for the textbook answer, which has to do with osmolarity, sodium concentration, or what have you.) The superficial capillary-deep loop vascular organization could be a clue to a guess; the thought process of getting to an answer is the sole interest:

> The deep vascular bed is embedded in the OVLT parenchyma, and lies within the brain, unlike the superficial bed, which is in the pial layer outside the brain. This suggests that blood-borne substances can easily penetrate into the brain parenchyma through the fenestrated endothelium of the OVLT. Furthermore,

the formation of glomerular tufts from the large caliber capillaries may cause stagnation of circulating blood. This would tend to promote the extravasation of the substances followed by their penetration into the brain (Yamaguchi et al., 1993).

The above, somewhat speculative excerpt was based on study in rabbits and rats (the glomerular tufts were found beyond the territory of loops, very close to the third ventricular surface). Duvernoy and Risold elaborate on the loops in a way that is relevant to Yamaguchi et al.'s tufts:

> . . . loops are always oriented toward the ventricular cavities, often coming almost up to the ventricular surface. These observations corroborate the hypothesis that specific molecular or physical interactions can take place . . .

One wants to say, "prove the hypothesis."

*

Fast forward to a study in rats, some years later:

> In contrast to the rostral pole of the OVLT, which interfaces the cisternal CSF . . ., the caudal pole of the OVLT interfaces the ventricular CSF through a thick layer of **tanycytes** [think: elongated, specialized ependymal cells]. Indeed, a multicellular layer of tanycytes formed the anterior wall of the third ventricle along the full extent of the BBB [blood brain barrier]-free zone. It has been proposed that tanycytes may serve as a physical barrier between the parenchyma of the OVLT and the third ventricle, an arrangement that would prevent bloodborne molecules diffusing into the OVLT from accessing the ventricular CSF. . . . Unlike capillaries outside the OVLT which are wrapped by astrocytic end-feet that contribute to the BBB, capillaries coursing with the OVLT were devoid of GFAP [glial fibrillary acidic protein] staining.

In contrast, these vessels appeared to be contacted by . . . processes arising from the tanycytes forming the rostral wall of the third ventricle (Prager-Khoutorsky and Bourque, 2015).

Whether the above is tantamount to proof, I won't say, but the anatomical relationships are interesting; moving from "outside" (pial surface) to "inside" (third ventricular surface), we have:

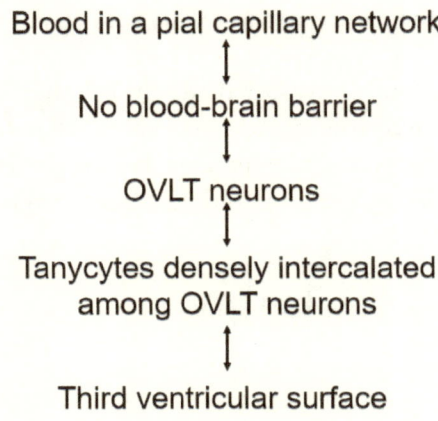

*

Let's ask the question once more: what does OVLT process, in terms of afferent data? Would you say:

    a. information about the external milieu,

or

    b. information about the internal milieu,

or

    c. information about two internal milieus (as revealed by both blood and CSF)?

I'm inclined to answer "c," but by doing so, I broach the perhaps too-philosophical question of what's outside vs. what's inside a brain.

*

Foregoing philosophy, one could more simply ask about OVLT's efferent connections, of which there are a few:

> . . . retrograde labeling studies have shown that OVLT neurons projecting to the [hypothalamic] supraoptic nucleus, ventrolateral periaqueductal gray, and ventrolateral preoptic area are concentrated within the dorsal cap [of OVLT], whereas those projecting to the bed nucleus of the stria terminalis are located in the [OVLT's] lateral margins (Prager-Khoutorsky and Bourque, 2015).

And, according to Johnson and Loewy (1990), there are other major efferents to paraventricular hypothalamic nucleus and the posterior pituitary, as studied in rats, never mind other possible projections to septum, dentate gyrus, cingulate cortex, and even the basal ganglia. Frankly, listing the efferents doesn't help me much beyond the acknowledgment of interconnection between sundry subcortical structures.

The real question is: what does OVLT sense . . . about us? The answer must be: aspects of the internal milieu as judged, perhaps, by a comparison between metrics of what's happening "inside."

24.

Wakefulness

Kinney et al. (1994) caused a bit of a nor'easter with publication of a neuropathology report in the case of Karen Ann Quinlan (she was originally named Mary Anne Monahan before adoption by the Quinlan family in 1955). Ms. Quinlan died on June 11, 1985 at the age of 31.

The storm evolved in ensuing correspondence to the *New England Journal of Medicine* that included a letter from California expressing "concern" about Kinney et al.'s methodology, one from Austria, one from New York, and one from a Colorado physician named Kaehny (Havton et al., 1994). The last prompted this reply from the editors: "Dr. Kaehny suggests, with tongue in cheek, that the article describing the neuropathological findings in the brain of Karen Ann Quinlan was out of place in the Journal. We understand his point of view, but we decided to publish the article because it was a carefully done study of an important case (ethically and legally, as well as medically), and the results were somewhat different from those that were expected."

Kaehny, it seems to me, had absolutely no tongue in his cheek: ". . . a headline report of a single case in an Original Article with superb anatomical description but little else hardly serves to enhance markedly our scientific knowledge of this entity," he wrote. And the editors, all tongues in their collective cheek, didn't really care to understand Kaehny's point of view, because the publication was a *fait accompli*.

A task-force report, published in the same issue as Kinney et al., 1994, identified one reason why the new pathologic study caused any tempest at all: "Relatively selective thalamic necrosis may also follow acute global ischemia, although the specific anatomical boundaries for this uncommon pattern have not been well described... (The Multi-Society Task Force on PVS [Persistent Vegetative State], 1994)." Previously, based on a reference cited by the Task Force, bilateral, *extensive*, thalamic neuronal loss, with sparing of brainstem and very modest cortical and hippocampal ischemic changes had been described pathologically only in an abstract regarding three patients with coma followed by a vegetative state after cardiac arrest (Relkin et al., 1990).

Someone said long ago that life would be but a stagnant pool without the occasional jarring interest. Kinney et al. provided an interest—earlier than 1994, in fact, because their findings had been presented in meetings at least two or so years prior to publication.

*

If wakefulness is familiar to all of us, why is its neural mechanism evasive?

> Although one can be asleep with the eyes open, or awake with the eyes closed, an individual with eyes that will open may be said to be awake, and therefore at least partially conscious. Put simply, an individual with eyes that will open is probably awake, and therefore at least partially conscious. Awareness refers to the collective thoughts and feelings of the individual and denotes the knowledge of one's own existence, sensations, and cognition in the external and internal worlds. The vegetative state refers to a state of wakefulness without demonstrable awareness, and thus raises basic questions about the nature of brain pathology which can lead to a dissociation of awareness from arousal (Kinney and Samuels, 1994).

That wakefulness doesn't mandate awareness deserves a brief comment.

*

Nieuwenhuys et al. (2008c) mention a "wake-promoting center" that we've visualized (see **Juxtallocortical Connection [to Hypothalamus]**") as a collection of histaminergic neurons in the vicinity of the mammillary bodies in hypothalamus. Those neurons project diffusely throughout both hemispheres probably under the influence of nuclei that project from the mesencephalic-pontine tegmentum. Brainstem input to hypothalamus is part of (it's the *extrathalamic* component of) an **ascending arousal system**.

Both in Kinney et al. (1994) and Relkin et al. (1990), absence of brainstem damage–essentially a normal entirety of brainstem (put to one side for a moment the question, raised in correspondence, whether Kinney et al. assessed cortex well enough)–was *a* reason for skeptical reception of the 1994 paper.

Twenty-five-plus years later, I think that attention has pivoted to the *thalamic* component of an ascending arousal system. One recent study, which we can examine in some detail, provides a sense of it (Ren et al., 2018). To be clear, "it" is the ***thalamic*** component of the ascending arousal system.

*

Ren et al. conducted a dozen or so experiments whose results can be edited and summarized. They studied mice; there were control groups in each of the experiments, including those introducing adeno-associated virus (AAV) into thalami.

1. They measured c-fos expression, which relates to recent neuronal depolarization, in paramedian thalamus. During a circadian awake cycle and, in addition, after extended wakefulness, they found higher c-fos specifically in paraventricular nucleus of thalamus (PVT) compared to other midline thalamic nuclei.
2. They interrogated PVT neurons further by injecting AAV into them. The AAV included genome to express a kind of calcium sensor. Calcium activity was higher during wakefulness than during sleep.
3. Next, to confirm PVT neuronal depolarization, they monitored with depth electrodes in freely behaving mice. PVT firing gradually decreased before sleep; in the transition from sleep to wakefulness, firing increased.
4. Since they used multichannel recording, they could temporally associate PVT firing with cortical activation. Increased PVT

firing happened about one second before cortical activation and about 1.5 seconds before behavioral arousal.
5. Again using AAV, this time with code for death of glutamatergic neurons by diphtheria toxin, they selectively ablated PVT. Neuronal demise happened about four weeks after injection. Afterwards, duration of wakefulness decreased; non-REM (non-rapid-eye-movement, henceforward NREM, as opposed to REM) sleep increased. (Multi-channel recording allowed for both EEG and EMG correlations.)
6. As a counterpoint to "chronic" death of PVT cells by way of the AAV vector mentioned in point 5, they also injected ibotenic acid for rapid ablation. Such lesioning caused fragmentation of wakefulness.
7. Next comes an optogenetic aspect, in several parts (points 7-10). AAV expressing channelrhodopsin, when injected into PVT, allowed them to switch PVT on and off by way of a directed light source. Optical stimulation of PVT's glutamatergic neurons during NREM sleep reliably induced wakefulness. It took about five seconds for the effect to take place. Mice in REM sleep also aroused after optical stimulation.
8. They activated PVT neurons in mice under isoflurane anesthesia, with EEG burst suppression as a marker of anesthetic depth. The timing went roughly as follows: a. isoflurane for 30 minutes; b. optical stimulation for a couple of seconds; c. then measurement of time to emerge from anesthesia. PVT activation resulted in shorter times to clear from anesthesia.
9. In "**Thalamocortex**" we discuss midline thalamic nuclei in general, among them PVT, as "higher order" centers; they project to layer 5 pyramidal neurons in diverse areas of isocortex. Ren et al. next looked for a "downstream" effect of selective PVT efferent stimulation (efferents to cortex), but:

> Together, our results do not sufficiently support a crucial role of the PVT-cortex pathway in controlling wakefulness. However, optical stimulation of the PVT-to-NAc projections [NAc: nucleus accumbens; see "*Nucleus accumbens septi*"] reliably elicited transitions to wakefulness from both NREM and REM sleep.

We'll wait a moment before comment on the above finding.

10. What about hypothalamic "upstream" input *to* PVT? (See "**Infundibulum**" regarding orexin-hypocretin neurotransmitters involved in both arousal and feeding; those two aspects of life are perforce related to each other: one doesn't eat a decent meal unless awake and aware.) Optical stimulation of lateral hypothalamus during NREM sleep increased the firing rate of PVT neurons; latency to a waking state from NREM and REM sleep decreased.

The authors concluded that PVT is both necessary and sufficient for the control of wakefulness, and that a lateral hypothalamic-to-PVT-to-nucleus accumbens pathway is also vital in that control.

*

The conscious content of wakefulness in a mouse is unknown, because we don't speak mouse. Control of wakefulness doesn't inform about awareness or, for that matter, about its absence in a vegetative state. Yet, something can be said in light of point 9 in the authors' run of experiments.

In "**Forebrain**, caudal" we allude to a thought that cortex may be driven by weak thalamocortical synapses (Bruno and Sakmann, 2006), though any input can be amplified, dampened, or otherwise modified depending on context (see also "**X and Y relay cells**"). What mitigates the surprise of point 9 is the "limbic-ness" of *nucleus accumbens septi*, olfactory tubercle, ventral striatum, and the striasomal system. If a mouse *learns* while awake, then the stage for its ongoing education is set by subcortex. To learn would seem to require awareness, even in the absence of human fluency in communicating with mice.

See "***Nucleus accumbens septi***," "**Olfactory tubercle**," and "**Projections of the Striasomal System**," and "**Quadrilateral Space of Broca**."

25.

X and Y relay cells

We've spent little time describing the morphologies of individual subcortical neurons. "Spine" is a word we associate with medium sized, densely spiny neurons of the striatum (see **Macro-, Microcircuitry**"), but there are also aspiny striatal neurons. A spine is an appendage of a neuron's dendrite. Aspiny neurons still have dendrites, just no overt density of spines. Aspects of dendrites can distinguish neuron types.

*

This chapter is about two types of thalamic projection neurons, which both have been extensively studied in feline lateral geniculate nucleus (LGN). Both types project to cortex–if you ask "which cortex?" I'll say "primary visual," but the visual cortic*es* are the subject of another monograph (See *The Visual Cortices*).

Called X and Y relay cells, the difference between them, most basically,[30] has to do with the look of their dendrites. In my discussion, I rely on two sources (Sherman and Koch, 1998 and Sherman, 2018), both of

---

[30] X and Y thalamic projection neurons–or "relay neurons," though "relay" has a somewhat problematic connotation–also earn their names because of upstream connections with different populations of retinal ganglion cells. We'll concentrate just on the two thalamic cell types. The problem with the word "relay" (a synonym for "projection") is the thought that nothing much happens when information transfers from the periphery (e.g., retina) to cortex. That view just isn't tenable.

which the interested reader should consult. My discussion will be absurdly basic by comparison.

*

While I enjoy and even love the etymologies of words, the association between "**dendrite**" (from the Greek *dendron*) and "tree" has always slightly confused me. I think of a tree with its trunk emerging from earth, with its branches in the sky, though dendrites can appear less like a whole tree, more like a fractal pattern; the arbor in the image, below, rather looks like a striatal spiny neuron:

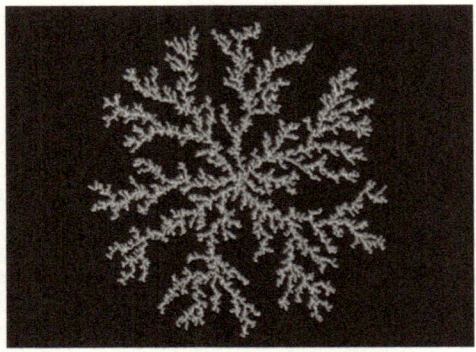

Full disclosure: the above *is* a fractal pattern, computer generated for the purpose of modeling a neuron. There's no soma or cell body; there are no axons as opposed to dendrites; it's just math in a graphic form.

Rather than visualize fractal complexity–for the record, however, X and Y cells have very intricate and wide dendritic arbors–, I'd think of a bipolar neuron cartoon, with one pole being its dendrite and the other its axon:

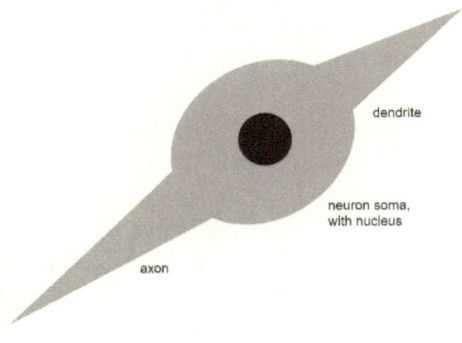

We know that both X and Y relay neurons of LGN receive retinal input and that they both project axons to cortex. Now we add more detail about input *at the level of the dendrite*:

> . . . the major information to be relayed is retinal, and yet this comprises only about 5% of the synaptic input. Although small in number anatomically, retinal input is nonetheless quite powerful in driving relay cells, and so we refer to this as the ***driver*** input. If the retinal driver input represents the main information to be relayed, what of the other nonretinal inputs? These have been lumped together as ***modulators***, because their main role seems to be to modulate retinogeniculate transmission. A modulatory role for nonglutamatergic (e.g., cholinergic, GABAergic, etc.) inputs is not surprising, but the point here is that many glutamatergic inputs (e.g., cortical) are also modulators, and only some (i.e., retinal) are drivers (author's italics, Sherman, 2018).

For the purpose of our discussion, the distinguishing aspect of driver input to LGN is that activates only ionotropic receptors at the relay cell.

A Y relay cell receives retinal driver (glutamatergic) input at its dendrite among other inputs, then its axon projects to cortex.

*An X relay cell receives retinal driver (glutamatergic) input at a specific lump along the dendrite, close to the neuronal soma (a "**glomerulus**," which unlike synaptic sites elsewhere in the brain is not sheathed by glial cells; synapses in a glomerulus are "naked"). X relay axons also project to cortex.*

I put a big capital "I" inside the glomerulus in the X relay cell, below, to remind myself that glomeruli have to do with *interneurons* as well as with retinal driver input.[31]

---

[31] Sherman and Koch (2008) elaborate: "Glomeruli seem to be related to interneurons, and it is interesting that the rat's VPL [ventral posterior lateral thalamic nucleus], which lacks interneurons . . ., also lacks glomeruli. . . . Glomeruli are common in other thalamic nuclei, but the pattern of specificity for functional types outside of the LGN is unknown." Sherman (2018) reiterates that glomeruli are "ubiquitous features of the thalamus, related to interneurons and found in most nuclei and species."

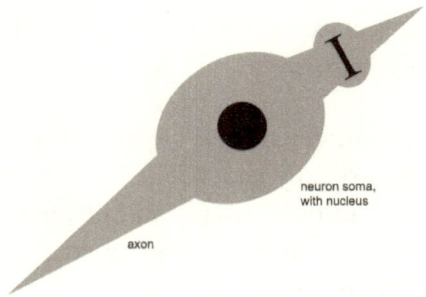

To oversimplify what happens inside a glomerulus in an X relay cell: 1. A retinal driver axon (glutamatergic) synapses at the proximal dendrite of an X cell; 2. A retinal driver axon (glutamatergic) also synapses at an interneuron dendrite (a modulatory interneuron and, let's say, it's GABAergic); 3. The interneuron also synapses at the proximal X-cell dendrite.

Driver input characteristically activates *only ionotropic* glutamate receptors (iGluRs) of relay cell dendrites, but the relay-cell-to-interneuron synapse (also glutamatergic) involves both iGluRs and metabotropic glutamate receptors (mGluRs).

> Activation of iGluRs typically occurs even at the lowest rates of afferent activity.... Activation of mGluRs usually requires higher rates of afferent activity, so the prediction is that, as the retinal input fires at higher levels, extra inhibition is brought to bear via the activation of mGluRs. Furthermore, this extra inhibition evoked by higher retinal activity would be long-lasting due to the prolonged effects of activation of mGluRs . . ..
>
> This overall effect, including its time course, seems an ideal neuronal substrate for the function of contrast adaptation [a bit later, we read more about the adaptation, which is an ability to decrease contrast sensitivity during epochs of high contrast and to increase contrast sensitivity during epochs of low contrast] (Sherman, 2018).

Sherman talks about "the prediction." Although there's data to support him, he's theorizing, and so can we. I think about the X relay cell doing what it does as the Y relay cell performs its less nuanced work at the same time. Y relay cells present cortex with a kind of raw(er) data set against which other input can be compared.

*

Either subcortex and particularly thalamus serve little real function (Sherman says thinking so would be absurd) or afferentation of cortex can be modified in ways suggested by anatomical aspects, like the lump or lack of one on a relay cell's dendrite.

26.

Zona incerta

The alphabet of this book started with *ansa lenticularis*, and it ends with a structure located near the ansa.

I don't know if the mistake is common, but one should be careful not to think that the region in question is something "inserted" somewhere. *Incerta*'s etymology doesn't relate to *inserere* (to "insert" in Latin), but rather to *an uncertainty*. August-Henri Forel, who first described *zona incerta* in 1877, admitted that nothing could be said about it with certainty at that time (Mitrofanis, 2005).

*

My interest in discussing *zona incerta* (ZI) has to do with what's inherently difficult when we study subcortex in general. The nut of our problem is found in this sentence (Mitrofanis, 2005): "[T]he connections of the ZI are very extensive, with projections being described with almost every center of the neuroaxis, from cerebral cortex to spinal cord." "*Very extensive*" causes even the strongest a weakness of the limbs. Nor is this helpful (the next sentence follows the one above): "Moreover, these projections are often bilateral, particularly with nuclei of the thalamus and brainstem." Does everything connect to everything in a brain?

Using ZI as an example, we can organize our learning without doing damage by oversimplification. Throughout this monograph, we've broadly used the method that I'm about to describe. Mainly, the tactic involves honest questions.

*

Where is ZI and what is ZI? We try to find an anatomic image, preferably one without undue magnification or some fastidious staining, but in the case of ZI, we default to a cartoon (see image in *"Ansa lenticularis"*). It seems to be a ventral continuation of the reticular nucleus of thalamus (see **"Reticular Nucleus of Thalamus"**) (Haubenberger and Hallett, 2018).

*

Is it a ventral continuation of the reticular nucleus of thalamus? (The question pertains to what it is.) Often, to answer the question of "what," it helps to retreat in time to the embryo or, alternatively, to consult other animal anatomies.

Here's Hayes et al. (2003) on the subject: "GABA neurons of ventral thalamus (reticular nucleus, ventral lateral geniculate nucleus, zona incerta, and nucleus of the fields of Forel) and of epithalamus appear at least 14 days before those intrinsic to dorsal thalamus [in the ferret, which is a kind of weasel]."

So, it's perhaps reasonable to think that ZI and reticular nucleus of thalamus, both being GABAergic, are related to each other as ventral thalamic structures. We have to be precise about what an embryological view of thalamus is, however. See **"Thalamocortex,"** in which we organize all 46 nuclei of a rat thalamus after editing *out* ventral thalamus and epithalamus, because fetal "dorsal" thalamus is what we consider the definitive structure in an adult rat (and adult human). Still reading Hayes, we learn about a belief (always a dangerous word in science) "that different classes of thalamic neurons are born more or less contemporaneously." The other shoe drops: "[n]ew studies now suggest that the pattern of development and glutamatergic cells of the mammalian thalamus is more complex."

*

Glutamatergic? OK, one now has to look around for evidence of a glutamatergic ZI, an example of which is the ZI projection to output basal ganglia nuclei, including *substantia nigra* (*pars compacta* and *pars reticulata*) and *globus pallidus* (Mitrofanis, 2005)–in apparent violation of a belief that output to thalamus from *globus pallidus* receives no return call from a thalamic structure (see **"Reticular Nucleus of Thalamus"**). Retrograde-anterograde monosynaptic tracing (Heise and Mitrofanis, 2004) and retrograde tracing (Gorbachevskaya, 2010) have been used to demonstrate the above ZI-"fugal" projection. For *substantia nigra* as an output structure, see **"Projections of the Striasomal System."**

*

So what? It never ceases to amaze what emerges from a literature search. For example:

> Let it therefore be suggested here, speculatively and tentatively, that the profuse and unusual connectivity of the zona incerta (or thalamus ventralis of non-mammals) allows it to perform the vertebrate brain's final conflict monitoring function, and that its internal global self-connectivity . . . serves to resolve whatever residual decision conflicts are left unresolved by other mechanisms (Merker, 2005).

I won't do justice to Merker's argument, which is lengthy.

The question whenever I read anything is: does my latest discovery (on PubMed, Google, or off my shelf) *help me*? It might or might not. That decision is mine or yours; the literature doesn't decide *for* either me or you.[32] Speaking as an anatomy-oriented person, after many years of reading anatomy and reading many other things, any "let it therefore be suggested" language makes me yearn to gaze wordlessly at a coronal section of brain, to glean what *it* can teach me.

*

---

[32] In *The Autocrat of the Breakfast Table*, Oliver Wendell Holmes, Sr. wrote about dead vs. living medical literature: "The dead is not all ancient, the live is not all modern" (quoted in Jones, 1985, p. 821).

See **"Claustrum"** for another instance (Crick and Koch, 2005) of authors talking about BIG ideas based on thinking about subcortex.

*

BIG is fine if you like BIG, but it's worth a moment to consider that much of what we know about subcortex has had to do with one, now-obsolete, retrograde technique ("obsolete" is Nauta's word, and the technique is his, too). A student of his nicely has this to say (Haber, 2016):

> Prior to the early [19]50's, only one stain was available to trace anterogradely labeled axons from their origin, the Marchi stain. This method stained specifically the degenerating myelin sheaths of myelinated fiber. Connections, therefore, could be determined solely from myelinated axons traced from well-placed lesions. However, the method did not identify unmyelinated or thinly myelinated axons. Moreover, the location of terminal fields could only be approximated. What was needed was a method that did not depend on the myelin, but rather the axons themselves. Nauta had set out in the 1950's to develop a stain that could identify the degenerating axoplasm by modifying the reduced silver methods of Bielchowsky and Cajal. The available stains were unable to distinguish between normal axons and degenerating ones. The Nauta method solved this problem of suppressing normal fibers unaffected by the lesion by using a weak solution of silver nitrate.

The bulk of this monograph is about what's been discovered by Nauta's backward-looking method.

There are those who, without much ado, have has influenced us subtly and permanently.

*

It's been observed that students find their teachers, not the other way around.

All worm holes find their students eventually, not the other way around.

Just ask a few questions, and read a bit.

You'll be found.

27.

The Themes of this Monograph

Items boldfaced in the preceding chapters indicate structures addressed in this monograph uniquely, though some might have been discussed in the prior five parts of this series. Believe it or not, I've tried to be parsimonious with my boldfacing in *Beneath the Cortical Surface*.

By chapter, in rough order of their appearance, let me list anatomical structures which we have encountered. Their number isn't too intimidating; and I won't include 46 nuclei (47, if you include *massa intermedia*) of the rat thalamus mentioned in **"Thalamocortex."**

*

A first theme to acknowledge is that all themes of this book relate to what a person can see with the relatively unaided eye. We allow ourselves cell-body and white-matter stains for a modicum of aid.

*

Ansa lenticularis

>medial *globus pallidus* or internal *globus pallidus*
>anterior and posterior commissures
>lentiform nucleus
>internal medullary lamina of *globus pallidus*

prerubral field (H): H either extends dorsally as Forel field H1 or ventrally as Forel field H2
fasciculus lenticularis or lenticular fasciculus (Forel field H2)
subthalamic nucleus of Luys
thalamic fasciculus (Forel field H1)
nucleus campi Foreli
prelemniscal radiation

Bed Nuclei of the *Stria Terminalis*

stria terminalis
terminal vein (superior, or anterior, thalamostriate vein)
septal nuclei
corticobasolateral amygdala
centromedial extended amygdala
extended amygdala (includes the bed nuclei of the *stria terminalis*)
periamygdaloid area

Claustrum

Diencephalon, embryology of

lamina terminalis
ventral thalamus (prethalamus)
dorsal thalamus
subthalamus
cortico-striatal-pallidal-thalamo-cortical organization
substantia nigra pars reticulata
entopeduncular nucleus
thalamic eminences or eminentia thalami
zona limitans intrathalamicus
external (or lateral) medullary lamina of thalamus
internal medullary lamina of thalamus
mid-diencephalic organizer

Eminences

> medial and lateral ganglionic eminences
> preoptic area, embryonic preoptic area

Forebrain, caudal

Globus Pallidus, lateral (in particular)

> *corpus striatum*
> caudate
> putamen
> *substantia nigra pars compacta*
> indirect pathway
> neostriatum or dorsal striatum

Habenula

> pineal gland
> *stria medullaris thalami*
> epithalamus
> *fasciculus retroflexus* or habenula-interpeduncular tract
> ventral tegmental area of Tsai
> raphe nuclei
> lateral and medial divisions of habenula

Infundibulum

> *tuber cinereum*
> supraoptic nucleus of hypothalamus
> paraventricular nucleus of hypothalamus
> suprachiasmatic nucleus of hypothalamus
> ventromedial nucleus of hypothalamus
> dorsomedial nucleus of hypothalamus
> arcuate nucleus of hypothalamus
> basal nuclei of Meynert (*nucleus basalis* of Meynert)
> lateral hypothalamic area

Juxtallocortical Connection (to Hypothalamus)

    periallocortex
    mesocortex
    fornix
    mammillary body
    mammillothalamic tract (of Vicq d'Azyr)
    posterior hypothalamus
    medial mammillary nucleus
    lateral mammillary nucleus
    tuberomammillary nucleus of hypothalamus
    lateral tuberal nucleus of hypothalamus (part of the lateral hypothalamic area)

Kern

Labeled Line

    primary motor cortex
    arcuate premotor area
    supplementary motor area
    area X of thalamus

Macro-, Microcircuitry

    medium-sized (not large), densely spiny neurons
    pyramidal tract type of corticostriatal projection neurons
    intratelencephalically projecting type of corticostriatal projection neurons
    direct pathway
    hyperdirect pathway
    pedunculopontine nucleus

Nucleus accumbens septi

    septum pellucidum
    rostrum of *corpus callosum*
    genu of *corpus callosum*

rostral body of *corpus callosum*
  caudatoputamen
  paleostriatum
  ventral striatum
  limbic striatum
  median forebrain bundle
  mesencephalic tegmentum
  orbitofrontal cortices

Olfactory Tubercle

  substantia innominata
  islands of Calleja
  olfactory bulb
  piriform cortex
  diagonal band of Broca
  locus ceruleus

Projections of the Striasomal System

  striasome
  matrix
  matrisome
  primary sensory cortex
  cingulate gyrus

Quadrilateral Space of Broca

  lateral olfactory stria
  horizontal limb of the diagonal band of Broca
  vertical limb of the diagonal band of Broca
  medial olfactory stria
  dentate gyrus
  cornu Ammonis
  anterior perforated substance
  interhemispheric fissure
  nucleus of the diagonal band of Broca

Reticular Nucleus of Thalamus

    internal capsule
    basal-ganglia-recipient thalamus

Sequences

Thalamocortex

    intralaminar thalamic nuclei
    midline thalamic nuclei
    first order thalamic nuclei
    mixed order thalamic nuclei
    higher order thalamic nuclei

Uncrossed?

Vascular Organ of the *Lamina Terminalis*

    organum vasculosum laminae terminalis
    preoptic arteries
    prechiasmatic cistern
    subcommisural organ
    area postrema
    tanycytes

Wakefulness

    extrathalamic component of the ascending arousal system
    thalamic component of the ascending arousal system

X and Y relay cells

    dendrite
    driver
    modulator
    X-cell glomerulus

Zona incerta

*

Two chapters describe a single anatomical structure ("**Claustrum**" and "*Zona incerta*").

Four chapters don't really introduce new anatomy ("**Forebrain, caudal**,""***Kern***," "**Sequences**," and "**Uncrossed?**)". We could use those four to help summarize themes addressed throughout the monograph.

*

"Gate" is a word traditionally used to describe thalamus, which is a conspicuous structure of caudal forebrain or diencephalon. "Gate" implies access, as in the original Anglo-Saxon sense of a "way to *get* in." A gate wouldn't be much of one if all passage across it happened without encumbrance. I broaden the sense of gates with talk in various places about channeling, volume control, aperture, or about the brain's *afferentation*, which includes more than information from peripheral sensory receptors.[33]

---

[33] S. Murray Sherman and R.W. Guillery go so far as to preface their *Exploring the Thalamus and Its Role in Cortical Function* (second edition) this way:

> In the past few years it has become clear that many and perhaps virtually all of the inputs to the thalamus are copies, through branching axons, of motor instructions. Some are motor instructions that are issued by ascending afferents, others are instructions issued by a lower cortical area and copied through an axonal branch via a thalamocortical link to higher cortical areas. That is, the information that the cortex receives from the thalamus is primarily information about ongoing motor instructions. Cortical functions, which have been analyzed in the past in terms of hierarchical links that carry sensory messages about external events, can instead be viewed in terms of corollary links, or efference copies that carry information about instructions for action, and these can be seen as providing the neural basis of perceptual processing (Sherman and Guillery, 2006).

By "lower" cortical center, they refer to cortex that receives sensory input, as

In Luria's spirit (Luria, 1973), I wonder about the many ways that cortex afferents itself. That the thalami, a gate to cortex, are themselves robustly innervated by cortex cannot be a matter of biological accident. Or, if it was a happenstance, it has proven to have survival benefit.

Without having cited either paper (yet), there can be no question that "Parallel Organization of Functionally Segregated Circuits Linking Basal Ganglia and Cortex" and "The Functional Anatomy of Basal Ganglia Disorders" have deeply influenced people who think about striatum and pallidum (Alexander et al., 1986 and Albin et al., 1989, respectively). As described in those still-vital papers, a *cortico-striatal-pallidal-thalamo-cortical organization*, I'd maintain, is an instance of cortico-cortical afferentation. And in thinking about that "loop" in its various manifestations, including (possibly) amygdalar connectivity, I've tended not to obsess over the relative contributions of the direct, indirect, and hyperdirect pathways. My reasoning has been, based on much work done since the late 1980's, that we would do well to understand first, and to a much better degree, the nuances of inhibition and excitation, because inhibition isn't always inhibitory (e.g., pallidal inhibition of thalamic nuclei) and because excitation (e.g., thalamocortical drive) may not "drive" as much as one might have once thought.

*

Ending the chapter "**Kern**" (German for a seed or nucleus) by stating the obvious, that cortical elaboration in evolution doesn't obviate nuclei, I refer, in part, to the efficiency of *Cajalian centralization*—that is, a concentration of cells—all cells related to each other, or perhaps all the same kind of cell—dealing with something that's distinguishable from something else. What's the "something"? The answer depends on the site. Hypothalamic nuclei, which are always hard to teach (but I try in this monograph), are impressively small, with enormously broad brushstrokes of effect. A relationship between appetite and arousal seems something that can't be doubted (I've never enjoyed a real meal on an actual plate while asleep). Both appetite and arousal have to do with lateral hypothalamus—I should

---

opposed to "higher" cortex that "connect[s] to motor actions or to memory storage." In terms of afferentation, however, both lower and higher cortex communicate with thalamus, as the authors have carefully described over the course of their careers.

say more precisely that they both have to do, at very least, with lateral hypothalamus and its posterior extension towards the mammillary bodies.

If we look just a bit dorsal to hypothalamus in the area of basal forebrain, we see nuclear-cortical interfaces that don't obviate Cajalian centralization. Rather, the centralization elaborates. After all, the brain as a whole, compared to the body, is a Cajalian centralization of function having to do with control of the body.

I myself believe (always a dangerous word in science) that there's a "greater limbic system" (Nieuwenhuys et al., 2008e), by virtue of which hypothalamus and many other (nuclear) structures impart valance to experience, or by virtue of which we remember what has happened in our lives. In light of what we learn about striasomes in *corpus striatum* and their "limbic-ness," it's not crazy to envision much of bilateral subcortex as part of a single, intricate system that Papez described when he wrote about "medial-wall" neural processing.

*

"**Sequences**" addresses birdsong and, if you will, the syntax and grammar of motion involved in how rodents traverse space. (I say "if you will" apologetically, because it's hard to suppress the syntax-and-grammar obsessed former English teacher in me.) "**Sequences**" is based on observations, albeit with the aid of various types of technology. And simple observation isn't quite a process of "murdering to dissect," as a poet once described the "meddling intellect." It's very neurological just to observe.

Certainly a theme in this monograph has been a focus on what we can actually see for ourselves–specifically *not* on those things that aren't quite visible which we're told to see (and then to learn by rote).

A dendritic arbor doesn't necessarily look like the tree in my back yard; instead, it can resemble a huge bush, a snowflake under magnification, . . . or an exercise, graphically depicted, in fractal geometry. A take-home lesson should be that, as someone has said somewhere, there are few straight lines seen in nature–whether in trees, bushes, or bolts of lightning in a summer storm. One wonders about the utility, heuristic though their intention almost always is, of wiring diagrams based on their myriad of straight-line connections.

Some years ago, Anne Graybiel, who influences much of what I write in these chapters, wrote a paper about the recoding of cortically derived information (Graybiel, 1998). Her own acknowledged influence in that publication is George Miller, whose 1956 paper is a delight, and whose discussion of recoding is as good as anyone's. I'll also mention that Miller often reads like a psychological information theorist, though I don't know whether he had been exposed to work (for example) by Claude Shannon (1948).

In any event, here's Miller on recoding:

> In my opinion the most customary kind of recoding that we do all the time is to translate into a verbal code. When there is a story or an argument or an idea that we want to remember, we usually try to rephrase it "in our own words." When we witness some event we want to remember, we make a verbal description of the event and then remember our verbalization. Upon recall we recreate by secondary elaboration the details that seem consistent with the particular verbal recoding we happen to have made (Miller, 1956).

The sequence (original story, rephrasing, memory storage, recreation by secondary elaboration in recall) assumes that the original story antedates any elaboration. In subcortical-cortical interactions, the temporal order seems more complex, insofar as cortex can lead or lag (for example) striatum. Or the neurons in both places can fire at that same time. Regardless, some translational activity seems inherent in cortical-subcortical communication. The recoding simply isn't a "relay," a word which implies that there's no change in information in a transmission. Recoding always introduces the possibility of change. As in information theory, it's possible to minimize the error rate in coding. Errors happen, so messages get re-sent due to noise. Context may require a need to change a first message–so, out goes another message. Some messages are too large to start, so they are recoded (think of what programs do to compress vast gigs of data into more manageable chunks).

*

In "**Uncrossed?**," I address whether subcortex on one side deals only with cortex on that same side of a whole brain. The answer isn't an unequivocal yes.

I do wonder about our common need to understand whether some pathway crosses or doesn't cross the vaunted midline. Such informational need–what we perceive as a need–is the result of our education: I've taught, for decades, about the importance of knowing where a tract (say, the lemniscal sensory system) crosses the midline, and I've congratulated myself when students, being students, parroted an answer, such as, "internal arcuate fibers of the low brainstem." "Good for you," I've said countless times to them. Yet, beyond basics, which are inevitably important in learning any trade, there's advanced consideration. Cajal called decussation a "singular phenomenon," because he was mystified by it. Even today, Cajal remains a tutor of the advanced student, whom all of us aspire to be.

The simple truth is that both crossing and non-crossing happen in nervous system architecture. When it comes to our "motor system" (for lack of a better term), I'd invite any student to revisit Peter Strick's work, and if she needs a single source with which to begin, I'd recommend Strick, 1985 or, perhaps even better (because it's earlier), Muakkassa and Strick, 1979. As discussed in "**Labeled Line**," injection of a retrograde tracer in primary motor cortex (in rhesus monkeys) resulted in labeling of more than homolateral cortex. Contralateral cortex (homotopic areas of contralateral cortex, to be specific) also labeled.

Other examples of unexpected contralateral connections can be found elsewhere in this book (see "**Claustrum**," or read about the "intratelencephalically projecting" type of corticospinal projections neurons in "**Macro-, Microcircuitry**," to cite just two instances).

The neurologist described in "**Uncrossed?**" isn't wrong when she contemplates in a "one hemisphere-one homolateral subcortex" organizational principle. But what are we all trying to understand, in the final analysis? Luria spoke of "the motor background" (also discussed in "**Uncrossed?**"), which, I think, is an amazing and practical concept. I move in space as a bipedal animal, as birds are bipedal, but maybe I'll head to work in the hospital. Or maybe I'll decide get to my desk to write more of these monographs. The motor background, for me, is the un-avian (because it's earth-bound) world of all things that I intend, plan, or very much want to accomplish. Does a "one hemisphere-one homolateral subcortex" view support an honest concept of what the background is? Anatomy is fate: we bihemispherically entertain our hopes and dreams.

REFERENCES

Page 3: Figure 1 (inset) from Haubenberger D and Hallett M. Essential tremor. *New England Journal of Medicine* 2018;378:1802-1810. Copyright 2018, Massachusetts Medical Society, reproduced with permission.

Page 7: The anatomical image (cellular, not fiber stain) is adapted from https://msu.edu/~brains/brains/human/coronal/1840_cell.html, and is used with permission from The Human Brain Atlas, part of the brain collections of the National Museum of Health and Medicine, Michigan State University, and the University of Wisconsin. These collections are available online at http://brainmuseum.org, http://brains.rad.msu.edu, and/or http://neurosciencelibrary.org, and are supported by the National Science Foundation and the National Institutes of Health.

Page 9: https://wellcomecollection.org/works/apv7nb3m/items?canvas=429&sierraId=b24989915-1&langCode=ger. Public domain.

Page 10: https://wellcomecollection.org/works/q5ghqt5k[.] Public domain.

Page 13: Figure 2 from Crick FC and Koch C. What is the function of the claustrum? *Philosophical Transactions of the Royal Society B* 2005;360:2171-1279. Copyright 2005, The Royal Society, reproduced and modified with permission.

Page 23 Page 23 Page 24: The same anatomical image, used three times in series, is adapted from https://msu.edu/~brains/brains/human/coronal/1680_fiber.html, and is used with permission from The Human

Brain Atlas, part of the brain collections of the National Museum of Health and Medicine, Michigan State University, and the University of Wisconsin. These collections are available online at http://brainmuseum.org, http://brains.rad.msu.edu, and/or http://neurosciencelibrary.org, and are supported by the National Science Foundation and the National Institutes of Health.

Page 33: The anatomical image is adapted from https://msu.edu/~brains/brains/human/coronal/2240_fiber.html, and is used with permission from The Human Brain Atlas, part of the brain collections of the National Museum of Health and Medicine, Michigan State University, and the University of Wisconsin. These collections are available online at http://brainmuseum.org, http://brains.rad.msu.edu, and/or http://neurosciencelibrary.org, and are supported by the National Science Foundation and the National Institutes of Health.

Page 34: The anatomical image is adapted from http://neurosciencelibrary.org/Specimens/PRIMATES/RHESUSMonkey/sections/1122rhes.jpg, and is used with permission from The Human Brain Atlas, part of the brain collections of the National Museum of Health and Medicine, Michigan State University, and the University of Wisconsin. These collections are available online at http://brainmuseum.org, http://brains.rad.msu.edu, and/or http://neurosciencelibrary.org, and are supported by the National Science Foundation and the National Institutes of Health.

Page 37: The anatomical image is adapted from https://msu.edu/~brains/brains/human/hypothalamus/3c.html, and is used with permission from The Human Brain Atlas, part of the brain collections of the National Museum of Health and Medicine, Michigan State University, and the University of Wisconsin. These collections are available online at http://brainmuseum.org, http://brains.rad.msu.edu, and/or http://neurosciencelibrary.org, and are supported by the National Science Foundation and the National Institutes of Health.

Page 37: The second anatomical image on this page is adapted from https://msu.edu/~brains/brains/human/hypothalamus/4c.html, and is used with permission from The Human Brain Atlas, part of the brain collections of the National Museum of Health and Medicine, Michigan State University, and the University of Wisconsin. These collections are available online at http://brainmuseum.org, http://brains.rad.msu.edu, and/or http://neurosciencelibrary.org, and are supported by the National Science Foundation and the National Institutes of Health.

Page 40: The anatomical image is adapted from https://msu.edu/~brains/brains/human/hypothalamus/6f.html, and is used with permission from The Human Brain Atlas, part of the brain collections of the National Museum of Health and Medicine, Michigan State University, and the University of Wisconsin. These collections are available online at http://brainmuseum.org, http://brains.rad.msu.edu, and/or http://neurosciencelibrary.org, and are supported by the National Science Foundation and the National Institutes of Health.

Page 41: The anatomical image is adapted from https://msu.edu/~brains/brains/human/hypothalamus/6c.html, and is used with permission from The Human Brain Atlas, part of the brain collections of the National Museum of Health and Medicine, Michigan State University, and the University of Wisconsin. These collections are available online at http://brainmuseum.org, http://brains.rad.msu.edu, and/or http://neurosciencelibrary.org, and are supported by the National Science Foundation and the National Institutes of Health.

Page 48: The anatomical image is adapted from http://neurosciencelibrary.org/specimens/primates/rhesusmonkey/brain/Rhesusmonk6.jpg, and is used with permission from The Human Brain Atlas, part of the brain collections of the National Museum of Health and Medicine, Michigan State University, and the University of Wisconsin. These collections are available online at http://brainmuseum.org, http://brains.rad.msu.edu, and/or http://neurosciencelibrary.org, and are supported by the National Science Foundation and the National Institutes of Health.

Page 57: The anatomical image is adapted from https://msu.edu/~brains/brains/human/coronal/1520_fiber.html, and is used with permission from The Human Brain Atlas, part of the brain collections of the National Museum of Health and Medicine, Michigan State University, and the University of Wisconsin. These collections are available online at http://brainmuseum.org, http://brains.rad.msu.edu, and/or http://neurosciencelibrary.org, and are supported by the National Science Foundation and the National Institutes of Health.

Page 61: The anatomical image is adapted from https://msu.edu/~brains/brains/human/sagittal/0512_fiber.html, and is used with permission from The Human Brain Atlas, part of the brain collections of the National Museum of Health and Medicine, Michigan State University, and the University of Wisconsin. These collections are available online at http://brainmuseum.org, http://brains.rad.msu.edu, and/or http://neurosciencelibrary.org, and are supported by the National Science Foundation and the National Institutes of Health.

Page 68: https://wellcomecollection.org/works/r6kzpkpr/items?canvas=430&sierraId=b28717752&langCode=fre. Public Domain.

Page 69 Page 70: The anatomical image (the second a magnification of the first) is adapted from http://neurosciencelibrary.org//Specimens/didelphimorphia/opossum/sections/fibersjpgs/opossum61-667F641Lg.jpg, and is used with permission from The Human Brain Atlas, part of the brain collections of the National Museum of Health and Medicine, Michigan State University, and the University of Wisconsin. These collections are available online at http://brainmuseum.org, http://brains.rad.msu.edu, and/or http://neurosciencelibrary.org, and are supported by the National Science Foundation and the National Institutes of Health.

Page 72: The anatomical image is adapted from http://neurosciencelibrary.org//Specimens/primates/owlmonkey/sections/444_OWLMONK_69-255.JPG, and is used with permission from The Human Brain Atlas, part of the brain collections of the National Museum of Health and Medicine, Michigan State University, and the University of Wisconsin. These collections are available online at http://brainmuseum.org, http://brains.rad.msu.edu, and/or http://neurosciencelibrary.org, and are supported by the National Science Foundation and the National Institutes of Health.

Page 104: Credit: Richard Wingate. Attribution 4.0 International (CC BY 4.0). Image available at https://wellcomecollection.org/works/p52x58bj/items?canvas=1[.]

*

Books and Monographs

Broca, Paul. *Mémoires sur le Cerveau de l'Homme et des Primates*. [contribution from Pozzi, S.], Paris: C. Reinwald, 1888. Available online at https://wellcomecollection.org/works/r6kzpkpr[.]

Burdach, Carl Friedrich. *Von Baue and Leben des Gehirns* [vol. 2]. Leipzig: Dy'sche Buchhandlung, 1822. Available online at https://wellcomecollection.org/works/apv7nb3m[.]

Carpenter, Malcolm B. and Sutin, Jerome. *Human Neuroanatomy* [8th ed.]. Baltimore and London: Williams and Wilkins, 1983.

Crosby, Elizabeth C. and Schnitzlein, H.N., eds. *Comparative Correlative Neuroanatomy of the Vertebrate Telencephalon*. New York: MacMillan, 1982.

Houk, James C., Davis, Joel L., Beiser, D.G., eds. *Models of Information Processing in the Basal Ganglia*. Cambridge and London: MIT Press, 1995.

Jones, Edward G. *The Thalamus* [facsimile edition in two volumes, originally published in New York by Plenum Press, 1985]. New York: Springer Science+Business Media, 1985.

Kahle, Werner. *Nervous System and Sensory Organs*. [3rd revised ed., trans. H.L. and A.D. Dayan, Volume 3 of Kahle W., Leonhardt H, Platzer W. *Color Atlas and Textbook of Human Anatomy*] Stuttgart and New York: Georg Thieme, 1986.

Longet, F-A. *Système Nerveux de L'Homme et des Animaux Vertébrés* [vol. 1]. Paris: Fortin, Masson et cie, 1842. Available online at https://wellcomecollection.org/works/q5ghqt5k[.]

Loewy, Arthur D. and Spyer, K. Michael, eds. *Central Regulation of Autonomic Functions*. New York and Oxford: Oxford University Press, 1990.

Luria, A.R. *The Working Brain. An Introduction to Neuropsychology*. Trans. Haigh, Basil. New York: BasicBooks, 1973.

Nauta, Walle J.H. and Feirtag, Michael. *Fundamental Neuroanatomy*. New York: W.H. Freeman, 1986.

Nieuwenhuys, Rudolf, Voogd, Jan, and van Huijzen, Christiaan. *The Human Central Nervous System* [4th ed.]. Berlin, Heidelberg, New York: Springer-Verlag, 2008.

Shepherd, Gordon M., ed. *The Synaptic Organization of the Brain* [4th ed.]. New York and Oxford: Oxford University Press, 1998.

Shepherd, Gordon M. and Grillner, Sten (eds.). *Handbook of Brain Microcircuits* [1st ed.]. Oxford and New York: Oxford University Press, 2010.

Shepherd, Gordon M. and Grillner, Sten (eds.). *Handbook of Brain Microcircuits* [2nd ed.]. Oxford and New York: Oxford University Press, 2018.

Sherman, S. Murray and Guillery, R.W. *Exploring the Thalamus and Its Role in Cortical Function* [2nd ed.]. Cambridge and London: MIT Press, 2006.

Swanson, Larry W. *Brain Architecture. Understanding the Basic Plan* [2nd ed.]. Oxford and New York: Oxford University Press, 2012.

*

Articles and Specific Chapters in Books

Albin RL, Young AB, Penney JB. The functional anatomy of basal ganglia disorders. *Trends in Neurosciences* 1989;12:366-375.

Alexander GE, DeLong MR, Strick PL. Parallel organization of functionally segregated circuits linking basal ganglia and cortex. *Annual Review of Neuroscience* 1986;9:357-381.

Alloway KD, Smith JB, Beauchemin KJ, Olson ML. Bilateral projections from rat MI whisker cortex to the neostriatum, thalamus, and claustrum: forebrain circuits for modulating whisking behavior. *Journal of Comparative Neurology* 2009;515:548-564.

Anderson SA, Marín O, Horn C, Jennings K, Rubenstein JLR. Distinct cortical migrations from the medial and lateral ganglionic eminences. *Development* 2001;128:353-363.

Bankiewicz KS, Oldfield EH, Chiueh CC, Doppman JL, Jacobowitz DM, Kopin IJ. Hemiparkinsonism in monkeys after unilateral internal carotid artery infusion of

1-methyl-4-phenyl-1,2,3,6-tetrahydropyridine (MPTP). *Life Sciences* 1986;39:7-16.

Bevan MD, Magill PJ, Terman D, Bolam JP, Wilson CJ. Move to the rhythm: oscillations in the subthalamic nucleus-external globus pallidus network. *Trends in Neurosciences* 2002;25:525-531.

Bolam JP. Microcircuits of the striatum. In: *Handbook of Brain Microcircuits* [1st ed.] Oxford and New York: Oxford University Press, 2010, pp. 109-119.

Borghei A, Cothran T, Brahimaj B, Sani S. Role of massa intermedia in human neurocognitive processing. *Brain Structure and Function* 2020;225:985-993.

Braak H, Del Tredici K, Bohl J, Bratzke H, Braak E. Pathological changes in the parahippocampal region in select non-Alzheimer's dementias. *Annals of the New York Academy of Sciences* 2000;911:221-239.

Brown SP, Mathur BN, Olsen SR, Luppi P-H, Bickford ME, Citri A. New breakthroughs in understanding the role of functional interactions between the neocortex and the claustrum. *Journal of Neuroscience* 2017;37:10877-10881.

Bruno RM and Sakmann B. Cortex is driven by weak but synchronously active thalamocortical synapses. *Science* 2006;312:1622-1627.

Cansler HL, Wright KN, Stetzik LA, Wesson DW. Neurochemical organization of the ventral striatum's olfactory tubercle. *Journal of Neurochemistry* 2020;152:425-448.

Carpenter MB and Peter P. Nigrostriatal and nigrothalamic fibers in the rhesus monkey. *Journal of Comparative Neurology* 1972;144:93-116

Carpenter MB and Sutin J. Olfactory pathways, hippocampal formation, and amygdala. In: *Human Neuroanatomy* [8th ed.]. Baltimore and London: Williams and Wilkins, 1983, pp. 612-642.

Consolazione A, Bentivoglio M, Goldstein M, Toffano G. Evidence for crossed catecholaminergic nigrostriatal projections by wheat germ agglutinin-horseradish peroxidase retrograde transport and tyrosine hydroxylase immunocytochemistry. *Brain Research* 1985:140-143.

Crick FC and Koch C. What is the function of the claustrum? *Philosophical Transactions of the Royal Society B* 2005;360:2171-1279.

Crittenden JR, Tilberg PW, Riad MH, Shima Y, Gerfen CR, Curry J, Housman DE, Nelson SB, Boyden ES, Graybiel AM. Striasome-dendron bouquets highlight a unique striatonigral circuit targeting dopamine containing neurons. *Proceedings of the National Academy of Sciences USA* 2016;113:11318-11323.

DeFelipe J and Jones EG. Neocortical microcircuits. In: *Handbook of Brain Microcircuits* [1st ed.]. Oxford and New York: Oxford University Press, 2010, pp. 5-14.

De Olmos JS and Heimer L. The concepts of the ventral striatopallidal system and extended amygdala. *Annals of the New York Academy of Sciences* 1999;877:1-32.

Douglas RJ and Martin KAC. Canonical cortical circuits. In: *Handbook of Brain Microcircuits* [1st ed.]. Oxford and New York: Oxford University Press, 2010, pp. 15-21.

Dum RP and Strick PL. The origin of corticospinal projections from the premotor areas in the frontal lobe. *Journal of Neuroscience* 1991;11:667-689.

Dumont EC. What is the bed nucleus of the stria terminalis? *Progress in Neuro-Psychopharmacology and Biological Psychiatry* 2009;33:1289-1290.

Ericson H, Blomqvist A, Köhler C. Origin of neuronal inputs to the region of the tuberomammillary nucleus of the rat brain. *Journal of Comparative Neurology* 1991;311:45-64.

Fame RN, MacDonald JL, Macklis JD. Development, specification, and diversity of callosal projections neurons. *Trends in Neurosciences* 2011;34:41-50.

Fraser S, Keynes R, Lumsden A. Segmentation in the chick embryo hindbrain is defined by cell lineage restrictions. *Nature* 1990;344:431-435.

Fuccillo M, Joyner AL, Fishell G. Morphogen to mitogen: the multiple roles of hedgehog signaling in vertebrate neural development. *Nature Reviews Neuroscience* 2006;7:772-783.

Fujii N and Graybiel AM. Time-varying covariance of neural activities recorded in striatum and frontal cortex as monkeys perform sequential-saccade tasks. *Proceedings of the National Academy of Sciences USA* 2005;102:9032-9037.

Gerfen CR, Staines WA, Fibiger HC, Arbuthnott GW. Crossed connections of the substantia nigra in the rat. *Journal of Comparative Neurology* 1982;207:283-303.

Gilbert MS. The early development of the human diencephalon. *Journal of Comparative Neurology* 1935;62:81-115.

Goldberg JH, Farries MA, Fee MS. Basal ganglia output to the thalamus: still a paradox. *Trends in Neurosciences* 2013;36:695-705.

Goldberg JH and Fee MS. A cortical motor nucleus drives the basal-ganglia recipient thalamus in singing birds. *Nature Neuroscience* 2012;15:620-627.

Goll Y, Atlan G, Citri A. Attention: the claustrum. *Trends in Neurosciences* 2015;38:486-495.

Gorbachevskaya AI. Organization of projections of the zona incerta of the diencephalon to pallidal structures in the dog brain. *Neuroscience and Behavioral Physiology* 2010;40:79-83.

Graybiel AM. The basal ganglia: learning new tricks and loving it. *Current Opinion in Neurobiology* 2005;15:638-644.

Graybiel AM. Templates for neural dynamics in the striatum: striasomes and matrisomes. In: *Handbook of Brain Microcircuits* [2nd ed.]. Oxford and New York: Oxford University Press, 2018, pp. 133-141.

Graybiel AM and Kimura M. Adaptive neural networks in the basal ganglia. In: *Models of Information Processing in the Basal Ganglia*. Cambridge and London: MIT Press, 1995, pp. 103-116.

Graybiel AM and Ragsdale CW. Histochemically distinct compartments in the striatum of human, monkey, and cat demonstrated by acetylthiocholinesterase staining. *Proceedings of the National Academy of Sciences USA* 1978;75:5723-5726.

Groenewegen HJ and Berendse HW. The specificity of the 'nonspecific' midline and intralaminar thalamic nuclei. *Trends in Neurosciences* 1994;17:52-57.

Hadjikhani N and Roland PE. Cross-modal transfer of information between the tactile and visual representations in the human brain. *Journal of Neuroscience* 1998;18:1072-1084.

Halassa MM and Acsády L. Thalamic inhibition: diverse source, diverse scales. *Trends in Neurosciences* 2016;39:680-693.

Haber S. Perspective on basal ganglia connections as described by Nauta and Mehler in 1966: where we were and how this paper effected where we are now. *Brain Research* 2016;1645:4-7.

Hamel EG. Telencephalon of marsupials. In: *Comparative Correlative Neuroanatomy of the Vertebrate Telencephalon*. New York: MacMillan, 1982, pp. 317-337.

Hardman CD, Henderson JM, Finelstein DI, Horne MK, Paxinos G, Halliday GM. Comparison of the basal ganglia in rats, marmosets, macaques, baboons, and humans: volume and neuronal numbers for the output, internal relay and striatal modulating nuclei. *Journal of Comparative Neurology* 2002;445:238-255.

Harman PJ and Carpenter MB. Volumetric comparisons of the basal ganglia of various primates including man. *Journal of Comparative Neurology* 1950;93:125-137.

Harris MC and Loewy AD. Neural regulation of vasopressin-containing hypothalamic neurons and the role of vasopressin in cardiovascular function. In: *Central Regulation of Autonomic Functions.* New York and Oxford: Oxford University Press, 1990, pp. 224-246.

Haubenberger D and Hallett M. Essential tremor. *New England Journal of Medicine* 2018;378:1802-1810.

Havton LA, Ohara PT, Jellinger KA, Jeret JS, Kaehny WD, Kinney HC, Korein J. Correspondence. The brain of Karen Ann Quinlan. *New England Journal of Medicine* 1994;331:1378-1380.

Hayes SG, Murray KD, Jones EG. Two epochs in the development of gamma-aminobutyric acidergic neurons in the ferret thalamus. *Journal of Comparative Neurology* 2003; 463:45-65.

Hazrati LN and Parent A. Contralateral pallidothalamic and pallidotegmental projections in primates: an anterograde and retrograde labeling study. *Brain Research* 1991;567:212-223.

Hedreen JC and DeLong MR. Organization of striatopallidal, striatonigral, and nigrostriatal projections in the Macaque. *Journal of Comparative Neurology* 1991;304:569-595.

Hegeman DJ, Hong ES, Hernández VM, Chan CS. The external globus pallidus: progress and perspectives. *European Journal of Neuroscience* 2016;43:1239-1265.

Heise CE and Mitrofanis J. Evidence for a glutamatergic projection from zona incerta to the basal ganglia in rats. *Journal of Comparative Neurology* 2004;468:482-495.

Hikosaka O. The habenula: from stress evasion to value-based decision-making. *Nature Reviews Neuroscience* 2010;11:503-513.

Hirata T, Li P, Lanuza GM, Cocas LA, Huntsman MM, Corbin JG. Identification of distinct telencephalic progenitor pools for neuronal diversity in the amygdala. *Nature Neuroscience* 2009;12:141-149.

Hnasko TS, Chuhma N, Zhang H, Goh GY, Sulzer D, Palmiter RD, Rayport S, Edwards RH. Vesicular glutamate transport promotes dopamine storage and glutamate corelease in vivo. *Neuron* 2010;65:643-656.

Hoover JE and Strick PL. Multiple output channels in the basal ganglia. *Science* 1993;259:819-821.

Innocenti GM, Dyrby TB, Andersen KW, Rouiller EM, Caminiti R. The crossed projection to the striatum in two species of monkey and in humans: behavioral and evolutionary significance. *Cerebral Cortex* 2017;27:3217-3230.

Jayaraman A. Anatomical evidence for cortical projections from the striatum in the cat. *Brain Research* 1980;195:29-36.

Jayaraman A. Topographic organization and morphology of peripallidal and pallidal cells projecting to the striatum in cats. *Brain Research* 1983;275:279-286.

Johnson AK and Loewy AD. Circumventricular organs and their role in visceral function. In: *Central Regulation of Autonomic Functions*. New York and Oxford: Oxford University Press, 1990, pp. 247-267.

Jones EG. The posterior complex of nuclei. In: *The Thalamus* [facsimile edition in two volumes, originally published in New York by Plenum Press, 1985]. New York: Springer Science+Business Media, 1985, pp. 573-604.

Kemp JM and Powell TPS. The cortico-striate projection in the monkey. *Brain* 1970;93:525-546.

Kiecker C and Lumsden A. Compartments and their boundaries in vertebrate brain development. *Nature Reviews Neuroscience* 2005;6:553-564.

Kinney HC, Brody BA, Kloman AS, Gilles FH. Sequence of central nervous system myelination in human infancy II. Patterns of myelination in autopsied infants. *Journal of Neuropathology and Experimental Neurology* 1988;47:217-234.

Kinney HC, Korein J, Panigrahy A, Dikkes P, Goode R. Neuropathological findings in the brain of Karen Ann Quinlan. *New England Journal of Medicine* 1994;330:1469-1475.

Kinney HC and Samuels MA. Neuropathology of the persistent vegetative state. A Review. *Journal of Neuropathology and Experimental Neurology* 1994;53:548-558.

Koutcherov Y, Mai JK, Paxinos G. Hypothalamus of the human fetus. *Journal of Chemical Neuroanatomy* 2003;26:253-270.

Krout KE, Belzer RE, Loewy AD. Brainstem projections to midline and intralaminar thalamic nuclei of the rat. *Journal of Comparative Neurology* 2002;448:53-101.

Künzle H. Bilateral projections from precentral motor cortex to the putamen and other pats of the basal ganglia. An autoradiographic study in *MACACA FASCICULARIS*. *Brain Research* 1975;88:195-209.

Lange H, Thörner G, Hopf A, Schröder KF. Morphometric studies of the neuropathological changes in choreatic diseases. *Journal of the Neurological Sciences* 1976;28:401-425.

Lansdell H and Davie JC. Mass intermedia: possible relation to intelligence. *Neuropsychologia* 1972;10:207-210.

Lim Y and Golden JA. Patterning the developing diencephalon. *Brain Research Reviews* 2007;53:17-26.

Luiten PGM, ter Horst GJ, Karst H, Steffens AB. The course of paraventricular hypothalamic efferents to autonomic structures in medulla and spinal cord. *Brain Research* 1985;329:374-378.

Luria AR. Movement and action. In: *The Working Brain. An Introduction to Neuropsychology*. New York: BasicBooks, 1973, pp. 245-255.

Marchand R. Histogenesis of the subthalamic nucleus. *Neuroscience* 1987;21:183-195.

Marín O and Rubenstein JLR. A long, remarkable journey: tangential migration in the telencephalon. *Nature Reviews Neuroscience* 2001;2:780-790.

Markowitz JE, Gillis WF, Beron CC, Neufeld SQ, Robertson K, Bhagat ND, Peterson RE, Peterson E, Hyun M, Linderman SW, Sabatini BL. The striatum organizes 3D behavior via moment-to-moment action selection. *Cell* 2018;174:1-15.

Markram H, Toledo-Rodriguez M, Wang Y, Silberberg G, Wu C. Interneurons of the neocortical inhibitory system. *Nature Reviews Neuroscience* 2004;5:793-807.

Martin-Bastida A, Lao-Kaim NP, Roussakis AA, Searle GE, Xing Y, Gunn RN, Schwarz ST, Barker RA, Auer DP, Piccini P. Relationship between neuromelanin and dopamine terminals within the Parkinson's nigrostriatal system. *Brain* 2019;142:2023-2036.

Masri R, Bezdudnaya T, Trageser JC, Keller A. Encoding of stimulus frequency and sensor motion in the posterior medial thalamic nucleus. *Journal of Neurophysiology* 2008;100:681-689.

Matsuda W, Furuta T, Nakamura KC, Hioki H, Fujiyama F, Arai R, Kaneko T. Single nigrostriatal dopaminergic neurons form widely spread and highly dense axonal arborizations in the neostriatum. *Journal of Neuroscience* 2009;29:444-453.

McCormick DA. Thalamocortical networks. In: *Handbook of Brain Microcircuits* [1st ed.]. Oxford and New York: Oxford University Press, 2010, pp. 87-97.

McDonald AJ. Is there an amygdala and how far does it extend? *Annals of the New York Academy of Sciences* 2003;985:1-21.

Medina L, Abellán A, Vicario A, Desfils E. Evolutionary and developmental contributions for understanding the organization of the basal ganglia. *Brain, Behavior and Evolution* 2014;83:112-125.

Middleton FA and Strick PL. Basal ganglia output and cognition: evidence from anatomical, behavioral, and clinical studies. *Brain and Cognition* 2000;42:183-200.

Miller GA. The magical number seven, plus or minus two: some limits on our capacity for processing information. *The Psychological Review* 1956;63:81-97.

Mink JW. The basal ganglia: focused selection and inhibition of competing motor programs. *Progress in Neurobiology* 1996;50:381-425.

Mink JW and Thach WT. Basal ganglia intrinsic circuits and their role in behavior. *Current Opinion in Neurobiology* 1993;3:950-957.

Mitrofanis J. Some certainty for the "zone of uncertainty"? Exploring the function of the zona incerta. *Neuroscience* 2005;130:1-15.

Muakkassa KF and Strick PL. Frontal lobe inputs to primate motor cortex: evidence for four somatotopically organized 'premotor' areas. *Brain Research* 1979;177:176-182.

Müller F and O'Rahilly R. The amygdaloid complex and the medial and lateral ventricular eminences in staged human embryos. *Journal of Anatomy* 2006;208:547-564.

Nambu A, Tokuno H, Takada M. Functional significance of the cortico-subthalamo-pallidal 'hyperdirect' pathway. *Neuroscience Research* 2002;43:111-117.

Nauta WJH and Mehler WR. Projections of the lentiform nucleus in the monkey. *Brain Research* 1966;1:3-42.

Nauta WJH and Feirtag M. Frontal sections. In: *Fundamental Neuroanatomy*. New York: W.H. Freeman, 1986, pp. 239-279.

Neudorfer C and Maarouf M. Neuroanatomical background and functional considerations for stereotactic interventions in the H fields of Forel. *Brain Structure and Function* 2018;223:17-30.

Nieuwenhuys R, Voogd J, van Huijzen C. Development. In: *The Human Central Nervous System* [4th ed.]. Berlin, Heidelberg, New York: Springer-Verlag, 2008a, pp. 5-66.

Nieuwenhuys R, Voogd J, van Huijzen C. Diencephalon: dorsal thalamus. In: *The Human Central Nervous System* [4th ed.]. Berlin, Heidelberg, New York: Springer-Verlag, 2008b, pp. 253-279.

Nieuwenhuys R, Voogd J, van Huijzen C. Telencephalon: basal ganglia. In: *The Human Central Nervous System* [4th ed.]. Berlin, Heidelberg, New York: Springer-Verlag, 2008c, pp. 427-489.

Nieuwenhuys R, Voogd J, van Huijzen C. Telencephalon: introduction and olfactory system. In: *The Human Central Nervous System* [4th ed.]. Berlin, Heidelberg, New York: Springer-Verlag, 2008d, pp. 337-359.

Nieuwenhuys R, Voogd J, van Huijzen C. The greater limbic system. In: *The Human Central Nervous System* [4th ed.]. Berlin, Heidelberg, New York: Springer-Verlag, 2008e, pp. 917-946.

Nóbrega-Pereira S, Gelman D, Bartolini G, Pla R, Pierani A, Marín. Origin and molecular specification of globus pallidus neurons. *Journal of Neuroscience* 2010;30:2824-2834.

Olsen GM and Witter MP. Posterior parietal cortex of the rat: architectural delineation and thalamic differentiation. *Journal of Comparative Neurology* 2016;524:3774-3809.

Olveczky BP, Andalman AS, Fee MS. Vocal experimentation in the juvenile songbird requires a basal ganglia circuit. *PLoS Biology* 2005:3:e153. https://doi.org/10.1371/journal.pbio.0030153

Oorschot DE. Total number of neurons in the neostriatal, pallidal, subthalamic, and substantia nigral nuclei of the rate basal ganglia: a stereological study using the Cavalieri and optical dissector methods. *Journal of Comparative Neurology* 1996;366:580-599.

Park A, Li Y, Masri R, Keller A. Presynaptic and extrasynaptic regulation of posterior nucleus of thalamus. *Journal of Neurophysiology* 2017;118:507-519.

Prager-Khoutorsky M and Bourque CW. Anatomical organization of the rat organum vasculosum laminae terminalis. *American Journal of Physiology. Regulatory, Integrative and Comparative Physiology* 2015;309:R324-R337.

Preuss TM and Goldman-Rakic PS. Crossed corticothalamic and thalamocortical connections of macaque prefrontal cortex. *Journal of Comparative Neurology* 1987;257:269-281.

Puelles L and Rubenstein JLR. Forebrain gene expression domains and the evolving prosomeric model. *Trends in Neurosciences* 2003;26:469-476.

Rakic P. A small step for the cell, a giant leap for mankind: a hypothesis of neocortical expansion during evolution. *Trends in Neurosciences* 1995;18:383-388.

Relkin NR, Petito CK, Plum F. Coma and the vegetative state associated with thalamic injury after cardiac arrest. *Annals of Neurology* 1990;28:221-222 [abstract].

Ren S, Wang Y, Yue F, Cheng X, Dang R, Qiao Q, Sun X, Li X, Jiang Q, Yao J, Qin, H, Wang G, Liao X, Gao D, Xia J, Zhang J, Hu B, Yan J, Wang Y, Xu M, Han Y, Tang X, Chen X, He C, Hu Z. The paraventricular thalamus is a critical thalamic area for wakefulness. *Science* 2018;362:429-434.

Robertshaw E, Matsumoto K, Lumsden A, Kiecker C. Irx3 and Pax6 establish differential competence for Shh-mediated induction of GABAergic and glutamatergic neurons of the thalamus. *Proceedings of the National Academy of Sciences USA* 2013;110:E3919-E3926.

Roland PE and Mortensen E. Somatosensory detection of microgeometry, macrogeometry and kinesthesia in man. *Brain Research Reviews* 1987;12:1-42.

Roper SD and Chaudhari N. Taste coding and feedforward/feedback signaling in taste buds. In: *Handbook of Brain Microcircuits* [2nd ed.]. Oxford and New York: Oxford University Press, 2018, pp. 379-388.

Sakai T, Mikami A, Suzuki J, Miyabe-Nishiwaki T, Matsui M, Tomonaga M, Hamada Y, Matsuzawa T, Okano H, Oishi K. Developmental trajectory of the corpus callosum from infancy to the juvenile stage: comparative MRI between chimpanzees and humans. *PLoS ONE* 2017;12:e0179624. https://doi.org/10.1371/journal.pone.0179624[.]

Saper CB. Hypothalamic connections with the cerebral cortex. *Progress in Brain Research* 2000;126:39-48.

Selden NR, Gitelman DR, Salamon-Murayama N, Parrish TB, Mesulam MM. Trajectories of cholinergic pathways within the cerebral hemispheres of the human brain. *Brain* 1998;121:2249-2257.

Sena E, Feistel K, Durand BC. An evolutionarily conserved network mediates development of the *zona limitans intrathalamica*, a sonic hedgehog-secreting caudal forebrain signaling center. *Journal of Developmental Biology* 2016;4/10.3390/jdb4040031[.]

Shannon CE. A mathematical theory of communication. *The Bell System Technology Journal* 1948;27;379-423 and 623-656.

Shepherd GM, Migliore M, Cavarretta F. Olfactory bulb. In: *Handbook of Brain Microcircuits* [2nd ed.]. Oxford and New York: Oxford University Press, 2018, pp. 309-322.

Sherman SM. Functioning of circuits connecting thalamus and cortex. *Comprehensive Physiology* 2017;7:713-739.

Sherman SM. Circuitry of the lateral geniculate nucleus. In: *Handbook of Brain Microcircuits* [2nd ed.]. Oxford and New York: Oxford University Press, 2018, pp. 87-98.

Sherman SM and Guillery RW. The role of the thalamus in the flow of information to the cortex. *Philosophical Transactions of the Royal Society B* 2002;357:1695-1708.

Sherman SM and Koch C. Thalamus. In: *The Synaptic Organization of the Brain* [4th ed.]. New York and Oxford: Oxford University Press, 1998, pp. 289-328.

Stepniewska I, Preuss TM, Kaas JH. Architectonic subdivisions of the motor thalamus of owl monkeys: Nissl, acetylcholinesterase, and cytochrome oxidase patterns. *Journal of Comparative Neurology* 1994;349:536-557.

Strick PL. How do the basal ganglia and cerebellum gain access to the cortical motor areas? *Behavioral Brain Research* 1985;18:107-123.

Swanson LW. The amygdala and its place in the cerebral hemisphere. *Annals of the New York Academy of Sciences* 2003;985:174-184.

Swanson LW. Centralization and symmetry. In: *Brain Architecture. Understanding the Basic Plan* [2nd ed.]. Oxford and New York: Oxford University Press, 2012a, pp. 43-56.

Swanson LW. The basic vertebrate plan. In: *Brain Architecture. Understanding the Basic Plan* [2nd ed.]. Oxford and New York: Oxford University Press, 2012b, pp. 57-88.

Swanson LW. The cognitive system. Thinking and voluntary control of behavior. In: *Brain Architecture. Understanding the Basic Plan* [2nd ed.]. Oxford and New York: Oxford University Press, 2012c, pp. 201-229.

Swanson LW. *Brain maps 4.0–Structure of the rat brain*: an open access atlas with global nervous system nomenclature ontology and flatmaps. *Journal of Comparative Neurology* 2018;526:935-943. For access to images: sites.google.com/view/the-neurome-project/brain-maps[.]

Swanson LW, Sporns O, Hahn JD. The network organization of rat intrathalamic macroconnections and a comparison with other forebrain divisions. *Proceedings of the National Academy of Sciences USA* 2019;116:13661-13669.

Switzer RC, Hill J, Heimer L. The globus pallidus and is rostroventral extension into the olfactory tubercle of the rat: a cyto- and chemoarchitectural study. *Neuroscience* 1982;7:1891-1904.

Takata N. Thalamic reticular nucleus in the thalamocortical loop. *Neuroscience Research* 2019, https://doi.org/10.1016/jneures.2019.12.004.

The Multi-Society Task Force on PVS. Medical aspects of the Persistent Vegetative State. *New England Journal of Medicine* 1994;330:1499-1508.

Thompson AM and Robertson RT. Organization of subcortical pathways for sensory projections to the limbic cortex I. Subcortical projections to the medial limbic cortex in the rat. *Journal of Comparative Neurology* 1987;265:175-188.

Tremblay L and Filion M. Responses of pallidal neurons to striatal stimulation in intact waking monkeys. *Brain Research* 1989;498:1-16.

Trujillo CM, Alonso A, Delgado AC, Damas C. The rostral and caudal boundaries of the diencephalon. *Brain Research Reviews* 2005;49:202-210.

Verney C, Zedevic N, Puelles L. Structure of longitudinal brain zones that provide the origin for the substantia nigra and ventral tegmental area in human embryos, as revealed by cytoarchitecture and tyrosine hydroxylase, calretinin, calbindin, and GABA immunoreactions. *Journal of Comparative Neurology* 2001:429:22-44.

Wilson CJ. Basal ganglia. In: *The Synaptic Organization of the Brain* [4th ed]. New York and Oxford: Oxford University Press, 1998, pp. 329-375.

Wilson CJ. Subthalamo-Pallidal Circuit. In: *Handbook of Brain Microcircuits* [1st ed.]. Oxford and New York: Oxford University Press, 2010, pp. 127-134.

Wulliman MF and Mueller T. Identification and morphogenesis of the eminentia thalami in the Zebrafish. *Journal of Comparative Neurology* 2004;471:37-48.

Yamaguchi K, Morimoto A, Murakami N. Organum vasculosum laminae terminalis (OVLT) in rabbit and rat: topographical studies. *Journal of Comparative Neurology* 1993;330:352-362.

Yin D, Valles FE, Fiandaca MS, Forsayeth J, Larson P, Starr P, Bankiewicz KS. Striatal volume differences between non-human and human primates. *Journal of Neuroscience Methods* 2009;176:200-205.

Zaborszky L and Gombkoto P. The cholinergic multicompartmental basal forebrain microcircuit. In: *Handbook of Brain Microcircuits* [2nd ed.]. Oxford and New York: Oxford University Press, 2018, pp. 163-183.

Zahm DS and Heimer L. The ventral striatopallidothalamic projection. III. Striatal cells of the olfactory tubercle establish direct synaptic connection with ventral pallidal cells projecting to the mediodorsal thalamus. *Brain Research* 1987;404:327-331.

Zhou N, Maire PS, Masterson SP, Bickford ME. The mouse pulvinar nucleus: organization of the tectorecipient zones. *Visual Neuroscience* 2017;34:E011. doi: 10.1017/S0952523817000050[.]

www.ingramcontent.com/pod-product-compliance
Lightning Source LLC
Chambersburg PA
CBHW020427220526
45464CB00002B/601